SPIRIT TALK

MINISA CRUMBO

SPIRIT TALK

a book of days

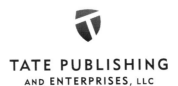

TATE PUBLISHING
AND ENTERPRISES, LLC

Published by Tate Publishing & Enterprises, LLC
127 E. Trade Center Terrace | Mustang, Oklahoma 73064 USA
1.888.361.9473 | www.tatepublishing.com

Tate Publishing is committed to excellence in the publishing industry. The company reflects the philosophy established by the founders, based on Psalm 68:11,
"The Lord gave the word and great was the company of those who published it."

Book design copyright © 2015 by Tate Publishing, LLC. All rights reserved.
Cover design by Gian Philipp Rufin
Interior design by Honeylette Pino

Published in the United States of America

ISBN: 978-1-63367-060-0
Health & Fitness / Alternative Therapies
15.03.27

to my family, friends and teachers

to MAMOGOSNAN, for all of the gifts

With special appreciation to my husband,
Jim Halsey.

Kiche Migwech, wewene kiche migwech

SPIRIT TALK

For all those left behind, caught out, fallen away, initiation deficient, wild Spirit seekers, lone wolf midnight prayer groaners, holy aspirants, and sweetgrass swingers…this book is dedicated to us. Where there is manure, there is a Spirit Horse to carry us and our fellow seekers on our earth walk and our star journey, so climb on and let's begin the ride to find the Spirit Fat with which to nourish our skinny and thirsting selves back to wholeness, balance, and harmony.

For we would remember: Our world was created in beauty, and it is beautiful still.

Dawn Woman

CONTENTS

Preface 15

Introduction.. 19

Artist Statement 25

Winter...Bbomgék: When the Year Begins 27

Quiet Time: The White Medicine Spirit Time—
    Firing the Seeds of Inspiration 27

Days 1–4 of Quiet Time: Are Spent in Silence 30

Day 5. Winter Quiet Time: When the
    Mother Earth Sleeps 32

Day 6. Gon...Snow Falls 32

Day 7. Firing the Seeds of Inspiration 33

The Original Instructions 34

Alignment 36

The Nature of Ceremony 37

Winter Solstice: December 21 41

The Listening Week.. 43

Negotiating the Listening Week into Spring:
    The Spring Marriage 47

The Book of Earth Days 48

Spring…Mnokmék.. 51

    Winds Carry Spirits to the Spirit World 51

    The Book of Earth Days, Spring..................................... 59

    The Winged Ones and Those Who Crawl

        Begin to Appear 62

    The Gratitude Principle 67

    Gratitude Principle Teaching, an Overview..................... 68

    The Gratitude Principle and the Sacred Right of Choice 70

    Color Vibrations, the Cradle and Web of Life................. 76

    Grounding Beauty 80

    Merging With Beauty, For Our Ears Only....................... 84

    Communication, Language, and Liberty 87

    Languaging, Hunting Happiness, and

        Grounding Beauty, Working Together...................... 92

Spring Equinox.. 93

    Cultivation of the Divine Inner Garden 95

SUMMER…Nibnek.. 117

    Revisit the White Plain, Wisdom Ancestor

        and Pure Spirit Lover of Innocence......................... 117

    Summer Arrives.. 119

    She Gives Away that New Life Might Come.................. 121

    Taking Off the Coats.. 122

    Summer Represents Undeniable Progressive Evolution

        and Unity with All of Creation................................ 123

    Birth: Visionary Separations and Creations.................... 125

    The Duality System 126

Summer Ceremonies: The Doctorings 127

First Steps 128

Dawn Woman Comes 129

New Life Comes 130

Good Medicines of the Body... 131

Good Medicines of the Mind and Spirit 131

Building, Shelving. and Initiating it............................... 132

Breathing and Being... 133

Knowing Beauty 135

Walking the Good Red Road 137

Scanning the Horizon 138

Early Autumn.. 140

Exploring the Essential Wildness of Life 141

The Good Red Road Establishes 143

Dawn @ the Ranch: The Summer Rains......................... 147

Building Trust, We Are Our Own Ancestors 149

Another Dawn @ the Ranch: Wild Roses
      and Santa Rosa Plums 155

Picking and Gathering for Balanced Health
      and Well-Being 156

The Broken Ground... 159

The Summer Solstice 163

The Summer Marriage Talks 164

The Summer Marriages 169

Summer—the Twenty-one Days Before Autumn Begins:
      The Autumnal Twilights Commence and the
      Thirteen Blue Corn Moons Measure Time 170

Our Seed Emerges with the First Harvest...................... 171

Autumn…Dgwagék.. 177
    The Autumn Harvest and the Fall Equinox.................. 177
    The Path of Light 178
    The Summer Sun's Medicine Face of Love
       and Trust and the Summer Sun's Medicine
       Face of Fear and Mistrust.. 179
    The Harvest and Picking "In a Good Way": Earth
       Ceremonies of the Gathered Plant, Leaf,
       Stem, Seed, and Root 188
    The Ceremony of Picking and Gathering
       "In a Good Way" 190
    The Direction of the West, the Physical,
       Medicine, and Introspection..................................... 191
    The World Tree of Life... 192
    Making New Relations.. 193
    Picking "in a Good Way".. 193

Harvest Recipes: For Feasting and Circle Gatherings 199
    Lillian Faye's Pecan Pralines 199
    Lillian's Lemon Pie.. 200
    Gram's Fried Chicken.. 201
    Grandmother Hogue's Wild Grape Dumplings............. 201
    The Circle Gathering, Part 1.. 203
    The Circle Gathering, Part 2.. 205
    The Circle Gathering, Part 3.. 206

The Circle Gathering, Part 4: The Spirit Plate,
    Alive in a Living World 208
Bringing It All Together 209
Formulating an Updated Brain Matrix 211

Fall Equinox 213
    Dawn @ the Ranch 214

Glossary 217
Suggested Readings 219

PREFACE

Bozho, ni je na? Hello, how are all of you?

This is the way it is with me, Minisa Crumbo Halsey, Citizen Band Potawatomi of the Shawnee, Oklahoma, agency and Muscogee Creek of the Okmulgee, Oklahoma, agency, this day.

In the way I was taught, or, "helped out" by my teacher, Marcellus Williams, Muskogee Creek, in Indian talk, everything of life, is ceremony. Therefore, life is always about remembering… for the old ones say, "It is not whether you will do 'it' but whether you will remember it." For at the core of our remembering, lives our sacred nature and the sacredness of all Creation.

I remember that my emergence point from the spirit world into physical form as a female two-legged was in the Kansas plains during the wartime winter. Now that time is long past and, as with any ceremonial venture, there is the prayer making, the leaving of the house, the beginning of the ritual, and a safe return to the same spot for the ritual ending. I offer thanks and credit for these circle realizations to another one of my treasured teachers, Martin Prechtel, that "big old orphan," as are most of us who are searching and seeking atonement and turn up at places like the Wisdom Keepers Gathering in Manhattan, Kansas.In the measured days of a workshop-sacred circle, we have shared carefully considered thoughts and council talk that the world might live.

My star journey eventually landed me in a home called Sweet Medicine land, and since that early morning my life has been one never, never far from the Mother Earth and Father Sky-Sun. This is always my/our birth, breath, sustenance, and source of endless beauty and wisdom. These are the things with which I would concern myself. I endeavor to invite, gift, and appeal to Spirit that a sacred circle be built, that all who enter might be able to purify and renew the heart, mind, body, and spirit. Then, may we most truly be able to live life "in a good way," to make a contribution that the children might live and to have some fun along the way...for all anyone truly wants is to be happy. Within the following remembrance and honoring circles are to be found and shared many proven and worthy tools to be taken forward into the larger circle of life.

To the Kansas plains we return...to remember that Mother Earth is the source of all true knowledge and wisdom. To her body we make ready the approach to the rivers, the winds, the rains, sleets, and snows, the bite of our father the Sky-Sun, and the Skebyak—the green beings. Let us make ready to come forward and to speak our names, bearing our gifts of wide smiles and tear-stained faces, hearts full of love and disappointment. And always, in the soul, may the perfect template of creation be remembered in silence, solitude, community gathering, and always in the first, last, and highest ceremony, that of remembering and of gratitude. For such is the required offering and price of being allowed to carry the gift of life in human form.

Come, let us gather and be for awhile of one mind.

Consider...honoring the Kansa Indians who came before us on this land, and petitioning them as ancestral spirits to receive our greetings and thanks and to look kindly upon us. We would walk softly upon the Mother Earth who supported their steps before ours and who will, with our prayers, support our steps and those of the seven generations who would come after.

That's the way it is with me.

—Wabaksekwe
—Dawn Woman

INTRODUCTION

Our relationship with Mother Earth, Father Sky-Sun, the Star Beings, and the Creator, "Master of all Breath," is what makes us feel like we have a right to live on the planet.

All wisdom and knowledge, the original teachings, arise out of these first, most beautiful and enduring gifts to us from the Creator. It is from these gifts that tradition, religion, and culture draw their inspiration, form, and practice. And it is in tracking the days and minding the breath through intention, form, and personal ceremony, as brought to us in the Medicine Wheel teachings and the natural world, that we find *Ways* to live and grow.

The best and only path we have toward the restoration, maintenance, and growth of our fullest potential—our sensitization to our place in the world—lies in rediscovering and grounding our highest intentions. Thereby, we begin to close our perceptions of separation with the Creator and to recognize and experience ourselves as seed co-creators, though our willingness to engage in Spirit Talks with our essential selves, our elemental parents, the Natural World, and the seasons.

Many helpers, systems, guides, messages, practices, religions, and traditions will be found that will provide essential assistance, inspiration, illumination, and core support on an individual's journeys toward, and within, the restoration and the continual renewal of balance and harmony. The culmination of these paths finds our natural destination within the unity path—the spiritual evolutionary path of humanity, which is drawn from and for the fullest honoring and manifestation of the Creative duality principle, now in place upon Mother Earth.

The unity path brings forward the most evolved and individuated gifts, of mind, heart, body, and spirit of the individual soul, to prepare us, in the highest and best possible way, for our successful launch as universal citizens.

The paths are many, but the first, most beautiful, enduring, and visibly tangible of the Creative gifts lie within and upon the wisdom libraries of the natural world, the ethers, our Grandmother the Moon, the Star Beings, our Mother the Earth and our Father the Sky-Sun, and all who live upon and within this miraculous world.

Be breathed and know life.

Aho!...and now, I'm going to go feast.

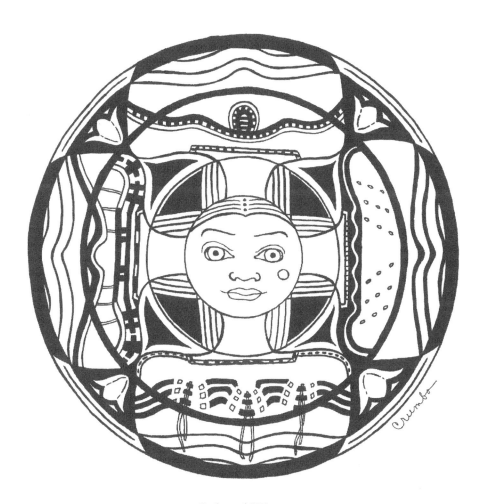

Beloved Woman

*To be painted with a red circle on the left cheek was, among certain peoples,
a most honoring and respecting sign. This painting honors
the many aspects of Woman.*

Beloved Woman
Minisa Crumbo

ALIVE IN A LIVING WORLD

This suite of thirteen black-and-white serigraphs presents a Native American perspective of the year, or thirteen moons, with months being measured and viewed by the passages of the twenty-eight day moon.

These images arise from my inner vision and experience as an artist within the context of Native American symbolism, myth, ceremony and art. Each image honors a facet of this beautiful world we were given to live in by the Creator—the first, last, most beautiful, and enduring gift from the Creator...

OUR WORLD WAS CREATED IN BEAUTY, AND IT IS BEAUTIFUL STILL

This beautiful creation of Mother Earth and Father Sky-Sun offers each of us an opportunity to walk, always, in balance and harmony by remembering them as our *elemental* parents. We remember...we have access to an orderly and supportive life view within the context of the Sun, Moon, seasons, the natural world, and the elementals of wind, earth, fire, water and the directions of the Medicine Wheel. Often when it seems we walk in separation from others, and even from ourselves, we have but to look about us at the day or season to see what is happening to us, in the moment, as reflected by the seasonal activity of light, wind, weather, time, and temperature of day or night. Thus, we maintain, or begin to move once more, into alignment or fine-attunement to be at one with life.

Universally, the traditional view of life is one of a sacred nature. Myriad helpers and companions accompany each person, and these helpers may be recognized through vision, dream, inspiration, or experience. Vision, dream, and inspiration are personal and vital connections to enhanced understanding, experience and attunement with the Spirit World. In this way, we honor ourselves as Sacred Beings and begin, or continue, to participate as co-creators in a living world. And so, we move in wholeness and beauty.

> *May we have a strong body*
> *May we have a good mind*
> *May we have a heart full of love*
> *And know no fear.*
> *Aho!*

—Minisa Crumbo

Of all the paths and choices and histories, the energetic pathways of the directions and elementals are the most real and vital—true paths of rubber-like energy. I think they are only found by mind-oriented persons who comprehend the true energetic, light components of the Medicine Wheel, sensitizing to them and then, through choice and discipline, making a transfer of their view of reality from that of what is visible to the eye to that of the felt and known planes, the planes of insubstantial essence—life force. We must choose vibrant feeling and knowing. Get to know and remember what it senses, looks like to the inner eye, and track it down to its places on the Medicine Wheel. And fuse, merge, again and again with the strips, rays, fibers, and channels of light. Release, choose, walk away. Choose to reject former static identifying habits, nests, and home places—the wallows and known places—in favor of newer, lighter habitats. Find places of being that are lighter and broader. Challenge yourself to run with nothing and be all by saying yes to light. *Yes! Yes! Yes!*

The older internal order will go on anchoring and reflecting the ongoing physical face with very little effort and will be enhanced by the reorientation to the light. Just make sure that once the light paths open up, and you know it, that some mental program stores it 24–7, making awareness and experience of the light never far from surface consciousness, making the full experience known, close and available, as soon as possible. Form new habits of association through remembering over and over again, linking the moments like beads on a string until they can be slipped over the head and worn. By linking life force with your individual DNA, new codes of being and doing will "make," adjust, and authentically shift, transforming your mind to reflect an effortless and moment-to-moment refinement of consciousness and empathetic connection.

Our thoughts are our reality. We must think better, smarter, longer, and deeper about ourselves, our world, and what we really want that to look, feel, and be like. Be it. Do it. Don't let up. There are probably not a lot of words, thoughts, or pictures of exactly what you want, but you *will* know what it *feels* like.

Hold yourself in trust. It's easy, really. It's very buoyant and light. It gives an unattached relevance to all things. And this is where I think I must depart the mental-energetic keyboard and merge with the light in the night.

Dawn Woman
Midnight @ the Ranch

ARTIST STATEMENT

ALIVE IN A LIVING WORLD

And when we took physical form, we wanted to know things and we began to want things to do. Work, play, and ceremony came into being…all the living arts. We began to make mighty, striving efforts to close the perceived (and, what a strong perception it can be) separation between the Creator and ourselves. And then, we find out that knowing and doing is good—very, very good—but still only a luscious and illusive stepping stone to the unity merge with who we really are, the Godhead ourselves.

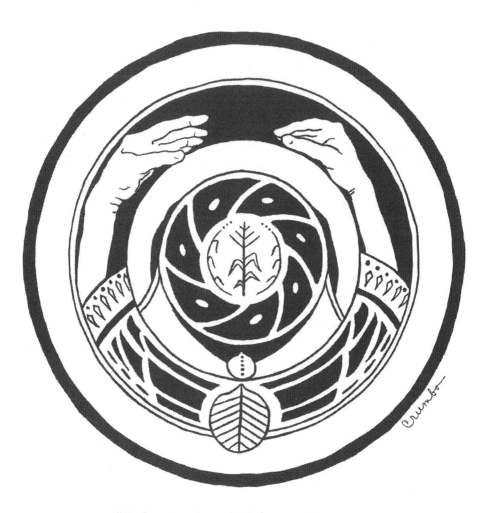

Mother Earth Holds Vision of New Life

The child within carries a dream of the Creative Forces to manifestation. Mother is both childbearing woman and old woman, her head and hair lines know wisdom of the evergreen tree and her garments speak of the flight of the winged ones. Her vision is at peace in her Sun-Moon home.

Mother Earth Holds Vision of New Life
Minisa Crumbo

WINTER...BBOMGÉK

When the Year Begins

What follows is the structure of a year that may be observed and considered to be a pattern by which to begin writing the new histories of a personal Book of Days as suggested by our elders and by interpreters of the Mayan calendar. From here, the sacred charge is for us to be writing the new calendars. Let us rise to the sacred charge in the full beauty and wisdom of our Holy Being.

We are not alone. There *are* proven and worthy tools and Ways.

Quiet Time

The White Medicine Spirit Time—
Firing the Seeds of Inspiration

DREAMING THE NEW GARDEN
IN THE QUIET RECESSES OF NOW

Now, at birth, all beings arrive with complete original instructions. Humans, in order to become fully and responsibly human, are the only species that must be taught appropriate socialization, kept sensitized to Spirit and the natural world, guided by wise example, and emotionally supported to adulthood. In the absence of strong role models or of an initiation tradition, we can and must do this by ourselves. In that case, we must turn to our bodies, minds, hearts and spirits, but especially the body. The next most trusted advisors and helpers for evidencing our original instructions are the Mother Earth, the Father Sky-Sun and the Grandmother Moon, guardian and protector of women. Much inspiration and wisdom may and can be drawn from studying the ways of these sentient and Spirit-filled beings of the natural world with whom we share breath and an Earth walk. So then, with acceptance, honor, and respect we remember the first gifts and call their names, as we now call our names: Beloved Woman and Beloved Man.

INITIATING THE CIRCLE OF SONG AND SINGING THE STORIES ALIVE

As the needle teeth of cold arrives, growth inducing and supportive fires of the previous seasons of harvest and summer and are concentrated, condensed, and drawn deeper into the seed-making union places. The Mother Earth cools her richness and invites all that live upon and within her body to burrow inward, toward our own inner fires and closer to her inner fires, stoking them with different fuels, fuels that woo the Grandfather Sky-Sun and Grandmother Fire Spirits with resonant hymns and melodious chants that speak of our peaceful and balanced intention that we might be viewed favorably and continue to warrant receiving their life-giving ways.

Breath is the first, most enduring, and then the final gift that greets us when we elect to emerge out of Spirit and to take physical form as a two-legged human being in the beautiful and challenging world of duality. It is by the ways of breath that we are breathed alive, receive information, and fuse into a *unified* person of mind, heart, body, and spirit...a sacred being. This sacred being we recognize ourselves to be is also the sacred that we recognize, or fail to recognize, in all living beings as a direct function of personal degrees of balance and harmony. The multifaceted and mutable faces of the natural world can be difficult to interpret, as difficult to accurately and positively interpret, at times, as our own or others' faces or truths. The Medicine Wheel Teachings have come down through time as a Way by which we might interpret and view these faces or truths, within the flexible and all accepting Circle of Life…another Web of Life.

A Circle gathering is good anytime, whether it is solitary, with only ourselves, or with others, because a circle is always strength and balance, and all living things have a place in the circle. It is now, the White Winter Medicine Circle time and we are prepared, whether we feel so or not, to recognize that by these inner teachings we have arrived at the place where we are "of one mind." Doesn't this feel good!

Let us now enter into the talking and listening Circle council. Let us take up the talking stick to show our original faces and speak our truths of how we would dream, find, fire, and anchor the good and sound seeds of life by which to live. Let us take up the talking stick and speak with the Creator and all who would witness, of the praise and gratitude that lives in our minds, hearts, bodies and Spirits, all ways, all days, from this time forward and forever more. *Aho!*

Let us now move into this ceremony. And how do we do this ceremony which we shall call the Firing the Seeds of Inspirition for the New Year Ceremony?

We begin by pausing to remember once again, that we are "being breathed" alive. We must prepare our purified and renewed truths and intentions to recognize and honor those seeds of inspiration which we would ask to come forward into the new year with us and, by our intention, we must "know and breath life" into those chosen seeds by sharing our breath.

SPIRIT TALK

These seeds may be named and their names spoken, but some will not. And some seeds, perhaps most, will be unknown to us at the present time. Some will sprout, some will not. It is largely out of our hands now as we pass our precious, blessed, and breathed seeds over to their own destinies and watch them manifest upon and within the sacred the Medicine Wheel of Life.

Days 1–4 of Quiet Time Are Spent in Silence

Day 5 of Quiet Time
December 6, 2013

THE TRUE NEW YEAR BEGINS AS WE INITIATE THE WINTER DREAM OF LIFE

Long before the first flakes fall here in the northern hemi-shell of Turtle Island, even as the shorter Sun loosens our stem connections and precipitates our spiraling drifts on autumn's winds, even as we make all of the seasonal returns, the collective memory of previous ancient creation stories and songs are gathered as a part of this year's harvest. The songs and stories are gathered along with the dried corn, hard squash, and dry beans, each carrying seeds, and within those seeds are their short and long lineage histories and creation stories. *So* many stories, for everything has a story and this is story time…

Long before the first flakes fall here in the northern hemisphere the turtle beings dig deep into some muddy bank to take their long winter naps within the sleeping body of the Mother Earth. The turtle beings and many others seek deep refuge not only within the Mother's body but also within her song…the heartbeat of her song. For our heartbeat and the heartbeat of the Mother Earth are one, and within the time of the winter Sun and the winter rest we are offered the organized cyclical return of the Medicine Wheel—the "white spirit medicine of the north."

As we remember these gifts, we also have the sacred charge to remember to recalibrate our heartbeat with the heartbeat of Mother Earth. We would also remember that her heartbeat pulses through and alongside the Father Sky-Sun's medicine planted within her body long ago, when the earth was young. And so, we would also remember and recharge the systemic fires, partnerships, and agreements of duality, as the duality principle faithfully and seasonally produces and reproduces the Creator's vision of life, as we know it now to be on Turtle Island.

This web of life, so carefully drawn, and for so long a time, is, at this moment or any moment in time, an aspect or a face of the Medicine Wheel. The Medicine Wheel represents the marriage of the prime duality concepts or Spirit gifts of the Mother Earth and the Father Sky-Sun. This fusion and partnership of Creative vision and energies may be viewed as the mothering and fathering that rose out of the vision of the Creator, or Master of all Breath, and gave physical form to life as we know it at this time. Our creation stories arise certainly from this time and before and beyond. Many of these stories are recounted in words or song, others within the touch of a hand, the look of a mouse, a passing cloud, shared laughter, wind on the water, wing song, a sob... so many are the stories of how we came to be. Let us now, in the "white medicine spirit time" create our own circle spaces within which to recount the myriad stories and myths—our personal and sacred creation stories. Let us dedicate time and attention toward honoring our own and all other's blood, sweat, and tears, as well as the dreams, visions, prayers and blessing works that go into our sacred Earth Walk as two-legged, full human beings.

SPIRIT TALK

Snow Woman comes...bringing the purifying power of the cold.

Day 5. Winter Quiet Time

When the Mother Earth Sleeps

Day 5 of Quiet Time
December 5, 2013, 16:13:55 CST

Now, is the time we two-leggeds may journey to rest, meet, and feed our deepest inner fires. At this time we make ready to petition the Grandfather Fire, son of the Sun, to help and guide us as we strive to fire the seeds of inspiration for yet another walk upon our beautiful Mother Earth, the beloved face of the Medicine Wheel of Life.

In this way we make ready to dream and prepare to birth our highest aspirations and prayers of living, always, "in a good way."

Begin to make ready, now.

Day 6. Gon...Snow Falls

Day 6 of Quiet Time
December 6, 2013, 20:35:12 CST

At this, and no other time, were these stories to be told. For now is when life is renewed by recounting the old stories, and the new myths are told. The new myths arise—fresh from experience— and our song or songs are made. Then we have songs to sing, for if the song face of tradition is not constantly changing, it runs the risk of becoming stale and outdated.

When the longer sun comes, our attention and movements are called out to participate in the renewed world, but now, "quiet time" is for the inner vision quest.

Day 7. Firing the Seeds of Inspiration

Day 7 of Quiet Time
December 7, 2013

Your song…

As you come to recognize your song-frequency, begin listening for the unceasing song-frequencies of every other thing. Each tree and species of tree has a unique song, the hissing and sizzling sound of the surf, the slow grinding sound that a mountain can make, the high-pitched ring of a tree. And as each element has its frequency, it also has a visible energetic emanation, which we call a "medicine." These emanations, or medicines, are often what we like or find repellent about an element. For instance, we may take a photograph, draw color inspiration, make a perfume from its essence, plant one in the yard, or even go back to school and take a degree in this medicine or entity essence.

Entity essence's frequencies and their emanations have been measured and photographed by scientific devices. They have long been visible and known to all other living things, and certainly to some two-leggeds with sensitized awareness beyond the commonly held parameters of what defines life and consciousness. Random experiences of heightened awareness have probably happened to everyone, but then ceased when their attention was returned to more commonly held definitions of reality. One way to reopen and expand awareness is by relocating and identifying a personal resonant vibrancy beacon within our unified spirit center, a beacon that signals initializing life forces. Now, we are on the track toward finding and hearing our personal song vibrance, our medicine, and that of others.

SPIRIT TALK

Building personal medicine is the means by which we can deepen inner communion, build and maintain conscious interactions with the natural world and, most importantly, begin to establish viable and trustworthy communication with the Creator, of which we are an inseparable aspect. That is not always so easy to do. Often, our most accessible links to the Creative Mind and our own creative mind is through the "first gifts" made to us, beginning as far back as when the firmaments were laid down, when light and sound breathed our world alive, and the time when Mother Earth and Father Sky-Sun came to this part of the cosmos to take physical form and participate in our commonly held dream of unity consciousness and its offspring, the duality twins. And then *we* came and were seated with a superbly designed body, a relatively conscious mind, a heart capable of caring for others besides ourselves, and the core center of Spirit, which is eternally seeking information about and reunification with Source.

The Original Instructions

Day 8 of Quiet Time
December 8, 2013, 13:53:39 CST

In considering the original instructions as we understand them to be, we should project all valued goals into the future and be willing to keep them in mind. Willingly work toward seeing these goals meet with appreciable success, beginning with the first harvests of freshly renewed and fired seeds of inspiration, enthusiasm, hope, endurance, and stability.

Now comes the work of setting these things we shall call the "original instructions" in place and tending them with attention and highest consciousness. All beings are born with a set of original instructions. The clear physical instructions with which we all arrive is heredity patterning. We, like all beings, contain, produce, and reproduce our adaptive potential to successfully meet a wide variety of growth conditions—from birth stresses, the vulnerabilities of youth, reproductive opportunities, sickness, old age, and transition activities.

Within our specific lineages are past histories, charting the major evolutionary shifts. Science and medicine are able to measure and evaluate current and future intelligence and data shifts, and now, even extend their reach to enter original seed packaging and to manipulate base genetic structure in order to legally claim ownership of the developed seed stock for profit in the field and the marketplace. The former seed stock contains and reproduces itself according to its original instructions, while genetically modified seed stock does not. We intend to follow the original instructions, as we know them to be, thereby putting an end to that which is not real. We choose to continue measuring our steps to meet and journey within the mystical outlines of the original instructions to the best of our ability.

Within this text, the major theme is: The original instructions, as revealed and made manifest in the Creator's first gift to us, the two-leggeds. The most beautiful and enduring gifts of the unknowable cosmos, within which lives and is breathed alive our Mother Earth, our Father Sky-Sun, our Grandmother Moon, the Star Beings, the cognizant and powerful elementals—Water, Fire, Wind, the Green Beings, the Directions, Spirit Helpers, all beings who live upon, above, and within this mighty gift, the Medicine Wheel of Life…*Ho, Mitakweasin,* my relations, I ask you to overlook any omissions or mistakes in this, the naming…there are so many, and I am still learning how to become and live as a complete human being.

And now, I will pause to think on these things.

Alignment

Day 9 of Quiet Time
December 9, 2013

Life is the management and maintenance of successive align-ments. Focus is a tool of the alignment concept. Spiritual align-ment is a very personal position point that does not depend on anyone or anything else. We are experts at alignment and it is a small, but potent shift to apply these talents to building the inter-nal spiritual structure. In order to do this, it is essential to consider and select areas of previous time and interest allocations that can be reorganized and shifted in order to create new and consecrated sacred inner planes of deep personal ceremonial connection.

We are experts at running our lives. Let's consider it possible to make a lateral shift and transfer these talents to building chakra alignments or other specialized, societal, or codified fields in the sacred inner chambers of the mind, heart, body, and spirit. Alignments that precede and underwrite more visible and commonly shared and organized ceremonial concepts, structures, directions, and colors and the shelving necessary to comprehend, receive, store, and retrieve them at will. The Medicine Wheel can be a very exacting and expansive experience of the mental and physical aspects of the entire being, *unless* the way has been prepared by a willing spirit. We need to be able and willing to entertain new ways and delve beneath the surface attractions of the Medicine Wheel to prepare in spirit, so as not to become over stimulated and attached to yet another beautiful and intelligent, yet compelling diagram of life.

The Nature of Ceremony

Day 10 of Quiet Time
Dec 10, 2013

We have spoken of many things. Now let us examine the nature of ceremony, whether it be personal or collective expression:

1. Any and all ceremonies arise from a place of personal excellence that is seeking connection and unification with Spirit.
2. All life is ceremony.
3. The rest is detail.

Let us step back now and examine the large and complex group ceremonies that most people are attracted to and familiar with: the dances; the Sweat Lodge ritual of purification and renewal; the Sacred Pipe, if this is in your tradition; the Medicine Wheel Teachings; vision quests; fasting; church and synagogue attendance; hunting, gathering, and other living skills. These ceremonies, rituals, skills, and accomplishments are among the largest and most substantial ceremonial "beads" with which we are likely craft objects of personal medicine. We then string these bead and seed essences on a metaphorical or literal medicine necklace, or place them into an attractive medicine pouch or bag with the hope that these medicines will keep, build, and grow for us, and that our power might grow, that life might get better, that prayers for a loved one will bear positive fruit. But often these things do not happen, because our medicines lack the essential psychological underpinning and grounding necessary to put these prayers and dreams together and blow life into them. These building steps are to be found in the inescapable baseline life experiences and first ceremonies that we all pass through, as the birth canal is cleared and we are *breathed alive,* we begin being taught about how life is and how to live it. This then, is the origin of ceremony: Life and breath fused with survival mechanisms, with beauty, the different families of blood, affinity, and the natural world, rites of passage, Spirit Talks with the Creator, ourselves, and others. This is such a complex blend. It becomes our life work to sort it all out and progressively "evolve to simplicity and unity."

We would speak now other ceremonies...of all other ceremonies, and about how to get into living experience and vital connection with them. Vital experiences that acknowledge the existence and living presence of ceremonial (life) qualities are present in every sacred moment—experiences that recognize and prepare the ground for the new sprouts. It is absolutely necessary that we recognize this in order to accurately, securely, and habitually place the "small" and routine ceremonies of daily life into their larger contexts of specific origin and function, in order to till our ground and prepare a place from which to grow, know, manifest, make new seed, and return seasonally into the Creative mind.

Recognizing that "all life as ceremony" is fundamental to all other awareness and growths. The First Ceremony is that of "being breathed." This cannot be emphasized strongly enough. Missing this point is a final and irrecoverable detriment to healthy growth. The being breathed teaching is a tool that, unidentified or mislaid, cannot be replaced. This occurrence is all the more tragic if the loss is not consciously or unconsciously known. Identification of being breathed remains one of the more valuable intentions and gifts of ceremony and is a connection that can be recovered and successfully integrated. This is cause for great gratitude. The connection of these individual and Creative life forces is a fundamental intention, appeal, and hopefully successful function of ceremony.

However, until the first ceremonial grounds (breath) are consciously and warily laid, there will be little to no permanent retention or access to larger and more complex ceremonial gains.

Stepping back into the first ceremony, being breathed, is to say to oneself, "How am I living? Can I truly say that in every moment I am conscious of being breathed alive by the Creator?" If this is not the case, then there are slim hopes of building the vibrant and sturdy edifice capable of supporting spiritual aspirations, connections, histories, stories, songs, and the other activities of a lifetime of movement upon and within the Medicine Wheel, the gifts of Creation, and the weight of our own life. It is through being breathed, not *taking* breath, that we find the potential to connect and merge with the Creative mind and experience oneness with all living things. These are the basic tools and gifts by which we cultivate the consciousness and awareness to build, understand, and experience our personal ceremony.

From here, let us endeavor to remember that all life is ceremony. Ceremony adds value and depth to everything. All things suggested in this book should be examined and viewed as ceremonies, not exercises.

We must speak accurately, in order to correctly chart the mental and physical findings and adjustments that arise out of the intelligence of breath:

The First Ceremony, being *breathed alive* is invoked.

Breathe.

Be.

Now, embark on your personal ceremony of *Being Breathed*.

That is all for today, day 10 of the Quiet Time.

WINTER SOLSTICE

December 21

By the calendar of the natural world, the winter solstice marks the ingress into the profound precincts of the deep Mother Earth Womb, the original confirmation point of all seed soul, sprout and rootlet growth. The days and nights of silent contemplation and Quiet Time observances have served to quiet the mind and prepare the body, much as a field is prepared to receive the new seed. Winter means that much of the northern hemi-turtle shell of this hemisphere is blanketed by the purifying powers of Snow Woman's gifts and freezes. The southern most regions of northern Turtle Island receive a warmer gaze and touch, but the Winter Medicine remains the same. The Sacred Hoop of the Medicine Wheel is in balanced reverse in the southern hemisphere. We live always within the Sacred Rainbow Hoop. This hoop of life is a threshold of all of the moments of the eternal present. The eternal present we now find ourselves within and contemplating is the first of the White Plains of Spirit, others will follow in succeeding seasons, each with basically the same purifying intent. The winter solstice, embedded within the purifying power of the cold, cloaked with the white plain of purity, located in and upon the wisdom body of the original gift, represents the core wisdom quality of winter. The emotional intelligence of these qualities joins with Spirit to be purified by the cold, much as the summer fires purify by golden heat. Both points, the terminal white heat points of the Good Red Road, which connects the north with south, wisdom with love, are Spirit conception and physical manifestation made visible. Conscious arrival and acquaintance with the Winter threshold of the Sacred Medicine Wheel Hoop of Life is a primal renewal experience, made ceremony. If this is a new concept to you, trust that you have entered into one of the most beautiful and comprehensive "systems" in this galaxy and beyond for containing, supporting, and interpreting life in a sacred way. Best wishes upon this journey. The winter solstice is a naturally occurring station within the year and, as such, has accrued a long history. The holy days, holidays, are usually grounded in natural phenomena that grew out of the Creative Mind and manifested in the first, most beautiful and enduring gifts of our Mother Earth, our Father Sky-Sun and the myriad of clustering entities we call the powers and fixtures of the natural world. Out of the mind of the Creator also came the understanding of sacred structure and function which shall henceforth be called the Medicine Wheel Teachings and of the Sacred Hoop of Life, in which we two-leggeds came to know life today, within the duality system. As we took physical form two things happened: One, we dearly wanted to understand and two, we wanted things to do. Many things arose and evolved into histories, myth, and culture. The specific Medicine Wheel Teachings and understandings were given to the people of Turtle Island. The teachings are nonjudgmental and, as such, offer a place for all things. The changing nature and variety of life ensures that the teachings remain fresh and always evolving, therefore the sacred charge may originate out of a specific culture of tradition but the individual experience is always a personal encounter with the Creator. Think now upon the bounty that the summer solstice represents. The winter solstice, by opposition and balance, represents the energetic origin point of the year. The quiet time has cleared essential time and space to approach life essence itself, to walk into the white plain with only the Spiritual core self, to *merge* and *be* one with the Mind of the Creator, as one comes forward to commemorate and celebrate the "firing of the seeds" ceremonies. In order for the face of tradition to remain true, fresh, and desirable it must always be open to change. This then, is the sacred charge: to bring oneself forward in all possible wholeness, mindfulness, and beauty, and to conceive of and design ceremonies of personal meaning, fulfilling the sacred charge to be happy and to enjoy life. This winter solstice is our time to unite with the natural word. Take these long nights to rest, tell stories, celebrate, and dream deeply of life before the stronger suns call us forward once again to grow and to labor. But for now, enter into and be one with the conceptual Return of the Light.

January 30, 2014, 22:32:47 CST

The Listening Week

In January we emerge out of December, the Quiet Time, and into the first week of January, the Listening Week.

CORE ENERGETICS

Our precious seeds, the initial elements of core energetics, have now been fired with inspiration for the year to come. This activity lends new meaning and content to the New Year's resolution as an activity that marks a very important advent of the new calendar year. The act of forming a New Year's resolution is basically one of gathering up one's precious seeds and endeavoring to make an intentional life contribution or ceremony honoring our inner seeds, and also honoring and acknowledging the possibly ungrounded and unsupported hopes of previous vows and resolutions—vows that we knew would soon be overridden, forgotten, and sapped of their already low level of anchored dynamic energy.

It is a sad and laughable thing, that hopeless and lost will and chance to live in a better way. With any failure of a New Year's resolution, yet another chapter of our personal creation story is possibly off to another spiritually shocking beginning. But, the story is hopeless and lost only for lack of focusing and grounding with the core energetics that birthed the desire for happiness or New Year's resolution in the first place.

The core energetics of the first gift that the Creator bestowed upon us all, are the Mother Earth and the Father Sky-Sun. By following the seasons that these ancients weave anew every moment, we encounter the very first and most enduring ceremonies of the personal home circle and a schoolhouse of abundant and trustworthy wisdom and knowledge. It is out of our worthy and anguished need, necessity, and desire to connect, merge, and bond with the source of life that we are able to successfully seek, forge, and, ultimately, to partner our own divine format as a co-creator within the format of the Life Force itself.

And how do we do that? Let's go back...back, or forward, to the New Year's resolution, going deep, deeper, and following its recent seat of origin to the place in our perfect mind, heart, body, or spirit from where it arose and sits, pulsing, living, being breathed, often without our notice. The resolution that wants to be happy. It never wants anything else, no matter which mask it wears as it waits to be noticed...as it waits for you to gather enough energy to make it happen this time.

To begin, we locate ourselves in the first month of the thirteen-moon calendar now. Now. Do it. Remembering? The first week of January we listened and were relatively quiet and probably heard nothing extraordinary, or perhaps we did. The week of listening is essentially designed to quiet us even further, to enhance awareness and deepen consciousness of the New Year, of the newly fired seeds of inspiration, and especially of the tender love seed of happiness, the love seed that perhaps we harbor fears of betraying through forgetfulness again. Ah, how sad we have been by apparently not being able to stand by ourselves and manifest our heart's desire, the most sacred and special sacrament, the secret and almost unknown, even to ourselves, sacred apparatus which makes us want to live—our personal belief platform upon which rests the possibility of building any and all cultural or personal belief systems. With this pure and solitary platform in place, our personal values will not need to struggle so hard to establish a foothold. Footholds, by which to initiate, explore, ground, root, and seek the nourishment necessary to feed and grow the inner sacred body, mind, heart, and spirit, the sacred twin born out of the duality and moving inexorably toward the unification at both and all elements.

And, at some time within the Listening Week the whole world will be purified.

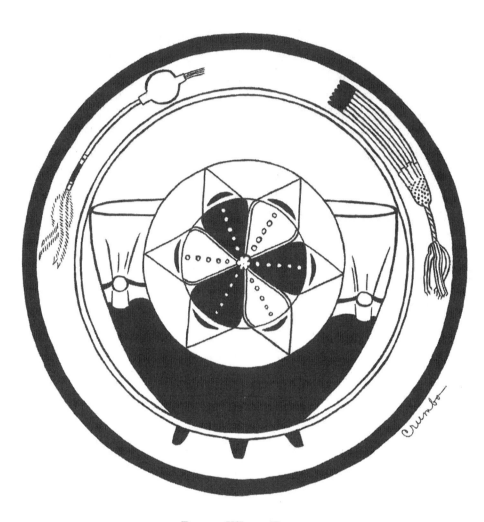

Peyote Water Drum

The Peyote Water Drum of the Native American Church rests within its
Sun and Moon, and speaks of the collective voice of Mankind raised
in a prayer of gratitude and thanks to the Creator.

Peyote Water Drum
Minisa Crumbo

Friday, January 31, 2014

Negotiating the Listening Week into Spring

The Spring Marriage

When the whole world is purified, so goes with it our mute personal ceremonies of intentional spiritual purification and renewal. And incorporated within this evolution to simplicity, within the innermost ground of belief potential, we become properly prepared to deposit our preciously prepared seeds within the Mother Earth and Father Sky-Sun marriage dynamic. This marriage dynamic, with the additional gift of our innermost seed selves, now becomes the renewed conception-marriage of our whole seed being, which draws close to unity with manifestation core energetics at its most complete, as close as we two-leggeds can now know it to be. It is the unity concept embedded within the concept of duality, the highest concept of marriage possible.

The marriage and merge into unity of our fired-seed intention with the core energetics of the Mother Earth, Father Sky-Sun, elementals, and directions is now set to participate in the renewed unfolding of seasonal brilliance and manifestation. Through recognition of these innate gifts and principles we decide, know or not know, feel, dream, breath, pray, dance, intuit, and miraculously construct the clearest and most personally balanced belief platform possible, from which to mount the next unfolding of the thirteen moons—our and all of Creation's most precious beings.

Now, we are readied to implicitly trust and to truly receive the life-giving properties of the wind, waters, moons, and stars, the energetic and informing downloads of the strengthening Sun's streaming pulses, of the Mother Earth, and the blessings of the Creator, Master of all Breath.

Migwech, wewene kiche migwech. Thank you, thank you very much.

—Dawn Woman

The Book of Earth Days

DECEMBER...QUIET TIME AND FIRING
THE SEEDS OF INTENTION

We have opened and visited the winter month we shall call the Quiet Time—December, the initial spot for this telling of a story of certain Earth days. We have remembered to count the harvest of the previous year's planting and gathering, we then selected those seeds of intention we found to be proven and worthy of being brought forward into the new year. We have thought on what those qualities are and what we would have them become.

Taking this intention and activity forward, we have summoned and invited the deep inner fires of the Mother Earth and the faraway fires of the Father Sky-Sun to sit with us and inculcate our selected seeds, hopes, prayers, and dreams with the power to grow, gratitude, and thanks, bringing them forward into the dreamed but yet unknown song of the new year.

We have rested and celebrated, told, thought, written, cried, sung, and danced our stories—our personal Creation stories. We have come forward and been counted.

JANUARY...THE LISTENING TIME
AND BRINGING THE UNFOLDING EMBRYOS
TO MEET THE SPRING

We have listened. We have made ourselves available for known or unknown purification and renewal blessings, passed through the uncertainties of the not-knowing time, felt the stirrings of

Spring as we arced the third week of January, and coupled not-knowing with hope and a deep unshakable certainty of life. That certainty has been buffeted by the rough winds of coming March and advancing spring. And then, with the Wind Beings as allies, we may have partnered with wind's medicine and shaken off the lingering slow releases of unwanted or unneeded histories through a sickness and getting well incident...all the while bravely marching our unfolding embryo songs forward to the beat of the big conductors, the Hall of Mother Earth and the warm Spirit Fire of Father Sky-Sun.

Through bravery, coaxing, remembering, and enduring, we move forward.

February 9, 15:41 CST

Patience, calm, and rest occur while residing in the Vision Quest cave, nestling deep within the accepting bosom of the Mother Earth.

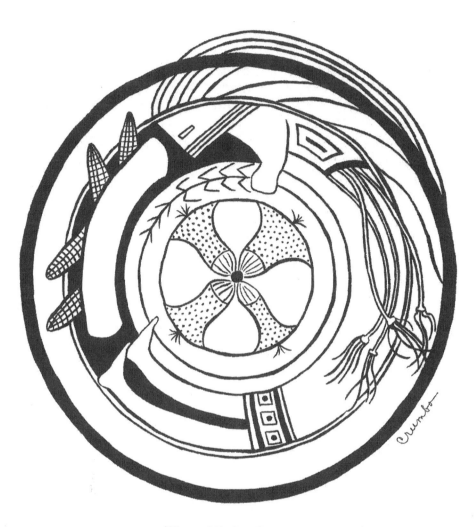

Moon Mother Emerges

*She emerges from the Dream of Creation, bringing forth a corn plant,
sacred symbol of life-giving forces. The Give-away from the plant people
that we may know life as human beings.*

Moon Mother Emerges
Minisa Crumbo

SPRING…*MNOKMÉK*

STILL RESTING, IN SILENCE

The people gather in spirit with magic food.

Winds Carry Spirits to the Spirit World

The winds of spring arrive to complete winter's work of finishing off anything that is revealed as dead, dying, and diseased, no longer wanted or needed. This is especially true for and visible with the tree beings, but holds true for everything else. This completing and carrying away time can be uncomfortable, but if we would remember to engage and merge with the Gratitude Principle, it will be easier. Do not expect to be comfortable in times of change, even times of the relatively benignly regarded season changes take on additional charges of importance and weight.

In spite of so many avenues open to the seeker, there still is no parallel or equal to regularly purifying or smudging oneself with sage and sweetgrass and then simply asking, "Great Spirit, what is going on here?" Then, listening and obeying.

The Grandfather Sky-Sun, unending and unceasing transmitter of the Creator's solar rays, and the heartbeat of Mother Earth remain, as the up above and the deep below of Creation, leaving us to discover ourselves as their sacred issue, and as potential energetic conduits of positive love and beauty without equal.

Everything is about everything.

February 18, at 20:55 CST

Greeting to the Sun

OUR CLOSEST RELATIONS

All of our relationships with the natural world have long roots, roots grounded in histories that long precede any given moment, and roots that comprise histories of their own, that might at any given moment be viewed as a cultural humus of the Mother Earth, hosting all sentient and nonsentient beings, and visiting energetics, vibrations, intentions, and influences; all interlacing, contracting and competing for the available mutable space and resources derived from solar energies emanating from and downloaded directly from the Source, Prime Creator, the Master of All Breath to us.

These relationships are agreements of a kinship and life exchange nature. We receive the solar fire and related intelligences to fuel our lives, while our acceptance, utilization, and expression (manifestation) of this energy through breath, movement, and inspiration produce a resonant exchange that nourishes our creative source in return. How this is identified, experienced, and socialized is an individual matter. Here we shall entertain and examine the individual solar equation as it interfaces with the core, life supporting units of planet Earth and its associated elements.

According to my tribal background, instruction, understanding, observation, and experience, the solar and earth elements shall continue to be put forward as living and sentient beings and as gifts arising out of the Creative Mind of one who shall henceforth be called the Master of All Breath.

THINGS TO THINK ON

Should you elect to observe and explore your life upon planet Earth within these given modalities, many opportunities will offer themselves as tools by which to discern, evaluate, and formulate; stage trials, build data banks through known and trusted avenues, be they intuitive or scientific; accrue personal data through the observance of seasonal movements, astronomy, or astrology, fasting, meditation or prayer, mathematics, the *Old Farmer's Almanac*, channeling; the "sight" or knowing; chance, teaching, theft, or trickery; vision questing in the men's or women's way; making love or war; the pangs of birth, and death, and change; eating; the quatrains of Nostradamus, the uncovered Sphinx feet, the Mayan calendar, or Medicine Wheel; the tarot; yoga, dance, or dream; the Dow, dinar, dollar, or yen; the Holy Bible, Holy Quran, scroll, cave painting, pecked rock, whale eye; or by measuring the winter hair of the wooly caterpillar. Whatever the avenue, if a thing exists, it is no secret. It may not be published or consciously known but it is woven into all of our being, and it is constantly changing at that, but it can be known because it *is*. The paths to knowledge and knowingness are as many, deep, diverse, mysterious, obvious, and rich as we, and many are the avenues. The challenge is to keep individual consciousness clear and open, so that the sought, obvious, or gifted knowledge does not unknowingly become altered as it passes through the filter of individual consciousness and personality.

These gifts and medicines, as well as the gifts and medicines of our elemental parents, the elements of the Medicine Wheel directions and colors; the Spirits of Wind, Water, Fire; the Green Beings, Stone Beings, and the medicines of their voices, songs, vibrations, resonances, and the messages of their very being are all key reunification passages. These beings *are* our relations. That is why when we kneel at the door of the sweat lodge we say, "to all my relations," because we remember the connections and would say so. That is why there is a noncompetitive place for all living things and concepts on the Medicine Wheel. That is why and how each of us is divinely fashioned to mirror truths for one another simply by being. In the rush, stresses, and necessities of daily life, these stupendous and gifted beings of the natural world are occasionally at risk of being either totally unknown, or even mistrusted, forgotten, or discounted, or uncomfortably outside heat and cold preferences…to our great detriment. The resultant losses and costs to soul placement and contentment, balanced mental health, feelings of worthiness and identity, and a vibrant physical "bag of bones" are well known.

Remembering these disparate elements and energies, healing, resting, and dreaming, and firing visions of the new year is a principal function of the White Winter Medicine Time. Listening to, reading of, or recounting old or new creation stories are the medicines by which we can originate, pollinate, and initiate a healthy, and increasingly aware, walk into the new year. What we have done, would do, and have done in the name of our precious seed brothers and sisters, we do for ourselves. These observances and ceremonies were enacted before us by our ancestors and shall be done by us. In this way, we participate in "keeping the world going."

The White Winter Spirit Medicine Time can be viewed as a safe or home zone where we can release, renew, and reset certain histories and motivations; relax, laugh, feast or fast, heal, and observe the building of our personal medicine as a Sacred Flowering Tree. This is done at leisure, but not necessarily alone. This *is* the main and appropriate activity for this season. For now, we are always seated at home, or possibly seated in the company and fellowship circle of our medicine brothers and sisters. We are prepared and willing to dream, breath our life into and grow the medicine seeds of the new year, by focusing on our loftiest ideals, intentions, prayers, blessing thoughts, gratitude, and loving kindness…with some assurance of success.

Please reread and study this section many times. If you elect to more fully honor the Quiet Time when the Mother rests and sleeps, consider eschewing superfluous movements and curbing the excessive use of machinery. Where possible, walk and use hand tools and limit electronic input. Speak less and more quietly...listen.

SPIRIT TALK

Moving onto and within the Medicine Wheel Teachings, in this seminal season, will support and assist your hopes and dreams of a more balanced and harmonious Earth walk, Beloved Two-Leggeds.

Aho!

Thursday, February 20th

The Marriage Refreshes

EMBRYOS AND INTENTIONS BEGIN
TO RAISE THEIR SONG

The Fire Beings and the Earth Beings...

Spring is an uneven time. Actually, it's all uneven, isn't it? However, the vagaries of the seeming unevenness, chaos, and change reveal power, medicine, and pattern when viewed in the context of the Medicine Wheel Teachings. If you are a visionary, dreamer, thinker, writer, business person, jeweler, singer, painter, or, name your own creative pursuit, it will be of value to note and chart, without endeavoring to process, our progresses and allow the medicines to reveal themselves throughout this, or any and all calendars of the thirteen moons, the twenty-eight day cycles of the Moon.

Spring is the bridge month that inexorably calls forth all embryos and fondly nursed creative intention. The full embryos tucked inside many large vegetable seeds, which formed via the pollen-laden leg hairs of bees, have been ready for a long time and only await favorable growing conditions to set out. They may wait hundreds of years or initiate new growth immediately. It all depends on the proper conditions of temperature and moisture and the agreement talks between the Mother Earth and the Father Sky-Sun. They have to remember and refresh their marriage story. A large part of their story has been counted and fed, all along, by other embryonic stories which have lain curled, secreted and quietly humming the potential and plans of their particular beauty and song.

Participation agreements are implicit as this song is orchestrated and the band is struck up. Rehearsals are ongoing. This part, no, *now!* You over there! But what about my solo? What? It's all solo…but done at the same time. Lots of new story-songs blast out a cacophony of slow and roaring starts, stimulating bird song to encourage and cheer the season along even as the winds tear at the new nests built for more new embryos. It is a rough passage.

The Wind-Breath Beings

The Wind Beings enter here to assist in carrying the fallen, dead, dying or diseased,…the no longer wanted or needed beings, who will not be moving forward into this new season. Yes, the Wind Beings carry spirits to the Spirit World and the new opportunities to be breathed alive into a living world.

The Wind Beings enter the big concert hall here, to take their place in the Song of Life as it strikes the initial chords at the fecund nods of the Mother Earth to the hot rays of the Father Sky-Sun. Consider taking and making daily time for initiating each new day, honoring and greeting the Father Sky-Sun by practicing a sunrise greeting ceremony.

The Sunrise Greeting Ceremony is universally present within all indigenous peoples' daily practice. There are so many solar honorings and practices. One is presented in this chapter. Consider incorporating a daily personal Grandfather Sky-Sun ceremony into your life, as an opening door into the sun-earth mysteries, by showing up daily. Upon welcoming the rising sun, or welcoming the sun at any time of day that you are awake and can make it. The ritual might proceed like this: First, I like to burn an offering of dry sage and sweetgrass, in that order, to purify the space and myself (sunrise has special pollen—new day healing energy). I speak the Grandfather Sky-Sun's name as I know it to be. I then begin to "make" prayers of gratitude and acceptance for my body and overall health. Secondly, I make prayers of gratitude and acceptance for the health and connection of my spirit. Thirdly, I make prayers of gratitude and acceptance for the physical health and well-being of the Holy Spirit in all things. Then, I bend down and touch the ground or deck, rise, and ask, "Grandfather, what would you have me know this day?"

Time has proven the wisdom of noting and accepting the first thoughts and visions and inspirations that come forward, no matter how simple or apparently insignificant they might appear to my mind. This is a time for acceptance and not interpretation, selection, or judgment. Now, live with this a bit and observe the knowledge and wisdom that it may hold for you,…not the least of which is agreeing and being willing to listen with complete trust.

GOOD MEDICINE FOR THE EYES

This sunrise ceremony has the power to instantly and painlessly burn away the thin layer of toxins that have risen to the surface of the eyes in the night. Pay close attention and you may "catch" this medicine in action. Many are the powers and gifts of the Grandfather Sky-Sun. *Aho!*

The Water Beings

The Water Beings enter here to bring life-giving moisture. Yes. We give thanks and recognition to these beings.

The Renewal

Enter here all of the named seed beings who have been remembered and called. All seed having been purified, returned to innocence—the not-knowing place, and then remembering their lives by dint of naked hope and aspiration, the rigors of what we shall remember here and call the month of January. January, that month so long ago and so full...that month of listening, of purification, that month of not knowing and then remembering. Finally then, sometime in the third week of the natural world calendar, comes spring and the long awaited seed-stirring time advances forward.

Spring, the one time among many, actually, when we can all renew, to see and experience the whole unfolding of the new songs. When the rigors of the first three weeks of January have been given their complete due and fealty, we may begin to see as a new being—once again a fresh and new being—as a child. Instead of carrying forward the full vision of the mature song, bringing forward few or no new verses, we now begin to find it possible to see, hear, taste, and know the absolute, unrehearsed new songs of everything, trusting that nothing of value or worth has been lost, and indeed, value has been added by the new songs.

The Medicine Wheel

The Wind Beings, the Water Beings, the Fire Beings and the Air Beings take renewed places in the East, the direction of the Medicine Wheel—the direction of the fire, young life, inspiration and illumination, whose shadow face is anger. Know all of these things and do not deny yourself the right to walk your walk and come to know all things that the Creator and your self would have you know. Know also that the true home of all beings lies at the center of the Medicine Wheel, where all paths cross, and the place where the Sacred Tree Flowers, us, make our home.

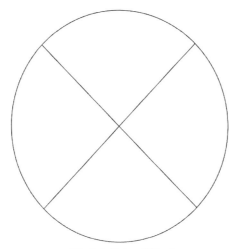

The Medicine Wheel
Minisa Crumbo

The Book of Earth Days, Spring

March, Diagramming a Personal Medicine Wheel, Part 1

And now, we respectfully begin to "make our prayers" of acknowledgement, gratitude, and thanksgiving as we approach and initiate our sacred intention of *being* "in a good way" through the proven and worthy ways of the Medicine Wheel Teachings, as they have come down to us through generations of loving, intelligent, and gentle medicine hands. It is a gift of knowing and understanding ways, of coming to understand and appreciate what it means to be a sacred two-legged in a very special way. It is with willingness and enthusiasm that we undertake to build life-fulfilling vision and the tools of understanding, resilience, flexibility, and strength to meet all times and conditions.

Begin to build a personal Medicine Wheel diagram on paper with a simple drawing.

Make a map of the Medicine Wheel design as you understand it to be and enter given facts and information on your life, facts and happenings from the time of beginning to read this Book of Earth Days, now, or in the opening months of December and January. Begin by entering your birthdate and mark the "Where We Are Now" section. Often people find that their position on the Medicine Wheel is not actually their physical birthdate, but instead it is the day when the Medicine Wheel Teachings were first presented. Just enter these things and study on them as time goes by.

The Winged Ones…Listening Again

The next spring birdcall you hear, raise your head back, open your mouth, and breathe in the next call. These are life-stimulating calls that the winged-ones offer in song, by which to vibrate life forward once again. These songs are life-giving gifts for each and every one of us. Accept them and think your gratitude to the bird people.

As the season progresses, notice that soon this song will not be sung any longer,…not until next year. This is their position, for now, on the Medicine Wheel. Enter it on yours. What kind and color of bird is it? What direction is it sitting in relation to you? Right, left, forward, behind, above? With yourself, the Sacred Being Who Approaches…entered both in the center and in the current month segment. Enter that.

Now that you have "caught" or been gifted with the appropriate frequencies of the season and have a winged one to enter, endeavor to "'carry'" this energetic and make a lateral transfer of this energy to initiate the construction of a rudimentary Medicine Wheel. Draw a circle and divide it into four equal segments or "directions" in the form of an X with a circle in the center, representing yourself in enduring alignment with the Sacred Flowering Tree. This may rest on a green ground or circle. The entire background can be blue, the color of Spirit. Now, color in the directions. The attendant qualities may be noted at the side, above, or below each direction. Construction paper, colored pencil, paint, fabric, leather, wood, metal, or another material at hand, or of choice, is acceptable and will speak of your personal choice and vibration.

The Medicine Wheel design may also be built on an altar cloth in the house, in a room where you can close the door, or built outside of stone or earth. If this becomes something to be thought on deeply, proceed to "make prayers" for an additional focus, on if this intention is to be pursued for construction on the floor or outside. If your aspiration appears to proceed forward unimpeded, prepare to smudge the would-be selected area well in advance of construction. Purchase some tobacco and mindfully approach the selected spot and "lay down," or offer, some tobacco or cornmeal to the Spirits of Place and make your prayers. Listen well and feel with full intention, as to whether this is an action to be followed through on or not. Listen and obey. If the answer is no, accept it with gratitude, acceptance, and love. If it is yes, accept it with gratitude and love, then sleep at least four nights on it before proceeding. Keep your medicine close and speak not of it, for now. We are making ourselves tuning forks of core energetics and building personal medicine. Let us be fully attentive and mindful in the most prayerful way we can assemble and put forward to Spirit. Everything depends on it.

THE COLORS AND DIRECTIONS

Color in these suggested directional colors. Later, you may establish personal alternate medicine colors of choice but for now these colors are broadly acceptable:

East	yellow	the mental plane	Fire
South	red	the emotional plane	Earth
West	black or dark blue	the medicine direction	Water

North   white   the direction of Spirit   Air
                              and the ethers

That is your start.

Letter from the Spirit Horse Ranch
February 20 at 17:02 CST

The Winged Ones
and Those Who Crawl Begin to Appear

As for us, here at the Spirit Horse Ranch, the winged ones, the
bird people are now being introduced as the first animal beings to
visit our local Medicine Wheel. They are seen and heard as they
appear in the direction of the east…Spring. In the house, the first
newcomers of the season have already made their appearances.
A grass spider laden with a heavy egg sac on her back appeared
on the bathroom floor. A fly buzzed in the house and a creaky,
dried-up scorpion was pointed out by one of the Beagles. All
were helped outside but for the fly, who flew away.

Many red birds are being seen and heard on the land. Today
they were here, as were crows, blue herons, wild turkeys, pileated
woodpeckers, jays, and another bird call that I recognize but
cannot put a name to.

It's been a day of tearing March winds and dropping
temperatures. Still, the Wind Beings tear away much dead,
diseased, and dying wood from the trees and carry it to the Spirit
World. I take it as a seasonal metaphor and willingly begin to
breathe out histories, thoughts, or attitudes that do not serve
me well, that are no longer wanted or needed, or that I elect to
no longer carry forward. It is a good time to ask the Sage and
Sweetgrass People to lend themselves to a "smudge" and ask them
to "help me out." *Migwech.*

For many of us who live in the Northern Hemisphere, March is the month where we just seem to go back and forth from the bedroom to the kitchen. It's too soon to plant anything, no mowing is needed, it's too soon to unwrap the pipes, but there are wonderful days in which to explore work and training, plan special projects, and to get the last long sleeps before the longer sun calls us out for another year.

March, Today, at 15:10 CST

The Medicine Wheel Construction, Part 2

BRAVERY, COAXING, AND REMEMBERING

If you are still present, read on. If you will, now study on these shaded and deeply personal words and qualities. If you continue to expand into and resonate with these words remember that the old people have said, "That which you recognize, you own." Introduce yourself by name, heart, need, and gently coax out the quality of bravery to join in your journey for awhile or forever.

These conceptual and energetic qualities can become among your most trusted friends and allies, when their inherent values are identified and fused with personal medicine intent. Personal medicine builds…These qualities will be of invaluable support and succor if you elect now, or at another time, to step deeper into the inner journey of the interconnected self, in a growing and vibrant connection to all the permutations of the Creative Mind.

The particular qualities of bravery, coaxing, and remembering, amongst many, will serve you well, as the uneven journey of life demands our fullest attention, our highest awareness, nimbleness of every sort, as well as willingness to come to know and then to measure accurately the steep heights and depths capable of being contained within this "sacred right of choice" world of spotty duality, and the innermost prize of unity consciousness. This is the Grail. Us, fully functioning in unity and duality, fed and nourished by the elixir of a balanced and whole Creative Mind, well and truly alive in a living world!

The Medicine Wheel Construction, Part 3

BRAVERY, COAXING, AND REMEMBERING

Following the prayer injunctions regarding a mindful approach to the Medicine Wheel Teachings and following the identification of suggested allied energetics, i.e., the Wind, Fire, Water, Stone Beings and others of personal value, we are now initially prepared to "initiate" our walk, beginning from the southeast boundary opening of the circle. Having previously gathered together an offering in spiritual, mental, or in physical form, from a number of things which you deem to be of the most personal value, lay the offering down. You are now as ready as you will ever be to approach and to enter the Medicine Wheel. Introduce yourself here by name and ask permission to enter the circle, petition to seek knowledge and sanctuary within the whole, and especially in the center, that place where the Sacred Tree flowers. It flowers, as a delicate and precious mist of unfolding potential, recognizing and fusing with life and understanding in all of its beauty, terrifying mystery, and blinding radiance of love. Bravery, coaxing, and remembering...

If and when the center is attained, sit or lie down and rest. This can and may be the most enduringly beautiful and secure place ever, within which to take up permanent identification and life... only time, remembering, and experience will reveal your personal truths regarding this place. There are many paths.

ACCRUING WISDOM AND KNOWLEDGE, AND RELEASING PERSONAL HISTORY

These messages float to the surface of my mind, heart, body, and spirit at this time of March. March, too soon to till and plant outside, but the appropriate time in which to bring forward those prepared and waiting seed embryos. The time to begin cultivating the Divine Inner Garden within, the spiritual twin and predecessor to the Divine Outer Garden of vegetable, office, family, relationship, friendship—be it the as the tender of small animals, kitchen, forge, or shop. These are the Divine inner and outer shops to get in order.

Wind is a friend of this order. When willingly worked with, the Wind Beings can be among the most powerful of allies as we endeavor to release and thereby purify personal history that is no longer, wanted or needed...dead, dying, or diseased. *Ay!*

BEING, DOING, AND REMEMBERING

Spiritual housekeeping depends on keeping the channels clear and the intent high and vibrant.

Spring, still indoor time for many, may include a time of sickness/wellness restoration. Maybe not...no worries... soldier on...

This an ideal time for a cleansing diet, revisiting exercise intentions, clearing household or office space of superfluous or outdated material, and making space for the new. The energetic pipeline, from deep, core source to high core source, can be addressed and plumbed to some, perhaps full, extent. It is possible that some material will be of a collective nature, not personal. This clearing will benefit the whole in a compassionate way.

As with much difficult or negative history, the holographic connections and cords may appear to be over and done with, invisible, as successfully managed as possible—sealed off or stored, forgotten or raw, or current. The connections can all be correctly addressed, but first, now it matters how they are handled; they continue to be present in memory hologram. This is the behind the scenes clearing that we are now getting down to—the deep energetic pattern cast by events, motives, history, DNA, Karma, intentions, thoughts, and actions. Actually, actions are the easiest to deal with because they can be "known" to a certain extent. The other things…it's really just a matter of willingness, intent, well-intentioned and skillful helpers, bravery and flat-out endurance to entertain these background and holographic ghost roots of mixed and clouded history. We successfully release these ghost roots by blowing their cover, by looking and seeing them, and then by releasing and sending them to their places of origin, or to return to the light energy pool, with gifts of love and gratitude. They cannot maintain for long, hidden in ascendancy or influence, when such a positive atmosphere is directed from one who would sit in the place where the Sacred Tree flowers!

This deep reach may extend even to tapping and releasing the primordial reptilian roots of certain levels of human development. The tapping of this level may reveal itself with tenderness or a "headache" at the base of the skull, the site of the latent and rudimentary root of reptilian record. There is no more reason to shrink from an encounter of this nature than any other, indeed there is more reason to clear our psyches of more of that dead, dying, or diseased and no longer wanted or needed material spoken of earlier. This is why the Wind Beings can be a powerful ally in this endeavor, particularly in this season when the field is being swept clear and prepared for the new. That is us! Fan yourself often with sage and sweet grass through times like these, drink a lot of water, do not dissipate, get as much good sleep as possible, prepare deeply nourishing meals of your choice, stay away from excesses of all kinds, and right your course as soon as possible. When the deviations do occur, and they will, do not beat yourself up or pass judgment on yourself, or any one or thing. Reposition yourself within the Medicine Wheel and remember who you are at your highest and best—a sacred being—and do not ever, ever forget this.

The light then has a chance to flow through us, with its vibrant and life-giving current from deep contact with the Mother Earth source and the Father Sky-Sun source, straight from the Creator, the Master of All Breath! May all life, wisdom, beauty, and the light of unending love be ours now and forever, from this day forward. It is good. It is very, very, good. *Aho!*

The blessings and gifts arising out of investigations of this nature *will* take time…but, we have time, don't we? Examine this thinking, perform your own tests, and accrue relevant data. If it feels good and works creatively, always creatively, I wish you well going into this new season as a blessed new, healthy being, and embryo of your highest self.

All has now been done that could have been done in order to prepare and celebrate the altar of coming New Life. So, when you first begin to comprehend these concepts, get out some metaphorical boards and nails, and hammer together some mental "shelving" upon which to place, store, remember, and *retrieve* this information and to carefully outline how the various engagements went. This too, is how personal medicine is built… being, doing, and remembering.

It is yours now, within which to live, explore, and celebrate.

The Gratitude Principle

The thirteen moons have been very busy and full with completion and initiation activities, and, as always, with the maintenance of that which has been integrated into our Eternal Present, the Now. For life is largely about maintenance…This past year I have completed a documentary on the life and artwork of our father, the Potawatomi Indian artist Woody Crumbo, as 2012 was his centennial year. This year has been about honoring family, friends, and heritage. Out of this time of honoring the ancestor has come this energy and vision. *Migwech.* Now, let us keep together for a while longer and speak on these things.

The "Walk" or "Sacred Path" put forward on these pages will support and honor our mysterious and precious selves. The Walk may be called, if you so choose, that of the Gratitude Principle. The path entries that follow may be read, spoken, sung, thought, studied, blogged, or journaled. This is the journey of your Sacred Self and your preparation begins with the walk within. In this way, we will have begun the work of "Becoming of One Mind" with one another for a while...the "Mind of Gratitude" for all of the gifts that the Creator has made available to us, the two-leggeds for this, our Earth walk.

Spring is an ideal time to dream the year ahead; pray, appeal, release, heal, renew, see and accept, planning and envisioning the new as we sit in the center of your Circle, recognizing partnership with our elemental parents, the strengthening Father Sky-Sun and the fragrant, warming Mother Earth. The spirit of the Gratitude Principle will give our hearts wings and sweeten our inner waters. For we remember: our world was created in beauty and it is beautiful still.

Come, let us walk together for awhile...

—Dawn Woman

Gratitude Principle Teaching, an Overview

This twenty-one-day period can be a personal planting of your inner garden—in any way you envision it—small or large. Mindfully, ask Spirit to give help with supportive garden needs, such as rain and sun on a spirit and physical level, whatever, and *however*, that might mean. Mainly, plant the perfect garden for yourself. Allow the volunteers from previous years to come up. During these twenty-one days, you will live and dream with your garden. It's fine not to know what to plant, for then Spirit will take you on a Spirit Journey. It could be a "do nothing garden," just a "being garden," like a Lily of the Field that neither spins nor toils. If you wish, you can sing, draw, paint, or write, etc., whatever is latent or developing within you. There is no wrong way to conduct this visionary garden—it can be a volunteer, or it may be in combination with what is physically planted. Allow yourself to gratefully observe what sprouts and grows, keeping the sprouts near, to grow along with you, wherever and *however* you go.

March 20 at 10:26 CST

THE GRATITUDE PRINCIPLE

The transformation, purification, and release of personal history and energy is the initial and principle medicine of the gratitude principle.

A posture of willingness to cultivate and adopt the habitual responses and thought patterns of gratitude and acceptance are the principle personal qualities we can bring with us into the Medicine Wheel walk. A posture of gratefulness helps to incorporate these qualities and tools, and that, once forged, will ultimately become internalized and utilized as medicine gifts during later times of active transformative experiences. Finally, the tempered tool of transformation emerges as us. We are the first change.

Yes, it will probably come as a full-out surprise to each of us that we, as solitary individuals, will not be fully able to effect many positive and enduring transformations without first undergoing this change of forging and living within a strong relationship with the Creator, Master of All Breath, one of whose faces happens to be the Medicine Wheel, as it represents and encompasses the myriad aspects of Creation. The journey continues…thou vision quester…thou sacred seeker of self and truth…thou who would be initiate of sacred and profane mysteries. Look no farther but look within, for the well of wisdom and scepter of knowledge are at hand when we shift into a renewed state of balance and harmony with the Creator, relinquishing all presumptions of isolating entitlement. True change of a transformative nature is a profoundly coordinated medicine event and, as such, can only begin to take place when we step up to the plate as unencumbered as possible by perceptions of division and separation. This is the secret of all true and good medicine. We are the first to be transformed...the true nature of initiation...to begin. It is good. It is very, very good...

We shall begin with choice as a sacred right.

March 18, 17:56 CST

The Gratitude Principle and the Sacred Right of Choice

The Gratitude Principle is, without a doubt, the most effective and enduring life tool I can pass on to you. Each of us is born with the sacred right of choice, and that knowledge is not always known. It is imperative that we recognize choice as a sacred right and observe how this medicine teaching can successfully fit in, merge, and empower both the Gratitude Principle and the Medicine Wheel Teachings. Without the understanding of these powers and gifts we risk living at the mercy of our own and others agendas, needs, and desires without clearly seeing that the give and take—choice as a sacred right medicine—belongs to all of us, be we plant, animal, or two legged.

This is a game changer. Without this tool and some understanding of how it works, we may lack the sufficient solid ground upon which to stand and build durable ethical models by which to live, view and interpret our own lives and those of others, and most interestingly, those of possible historical interest and instruction.

Two important medicines have been introduced here: gratitude and choice. They can and have been viewed separately. But I am challenged to walk in them together for they cannot ever, nor should they ever be asked to, live separately. They arrive together with us at birth and then, for many of us, fall precipitously and invisibly into the employ of survival and fulfillment tools, bids for attention, recognition and satisfaction...sometimes for a very long time—a lifetime. When this happens, life does not always make full sense. When these medicine gifts are not recognized and honored by look, word, or example we lose out... become lost. Who are we? Who are our people? Who are others? Social dysfunctions begin to take form when things do not happen as well as when things *do* happen. To suffer the unavailability of such important medicines as choice and gratitude is to be denied, neglected, or struck at the very root of ones personally developing self-knowledge and empowerment. To function, or to necessarily function, outside the grace of medicine recognition, meaningful personal ritual, and ceremony within the seasonal natural world and to suffer any diminishment, distortion, or loss of these valuable and intelligent interactive social tools is to sustain a blow struck at life itself.

But recovery is possible, because we are always in the process of becoming. "Being breathed" is one *half-life* breath and the exhale is a transition or release breath. We know life and we know death-transition...and we know continuance. Through breath, we know balance and imbalance, alternately. We live with an unshakeable knowledge of and trust in the continuance of life. This is where we start. Beginning again is built into the very fiber of our being. The knowledge, awareness, and practice of the Gratitude Principle and the mutual right of choice, in a given context of the natural world, positions us within both a starting point and a renewing platform.

This may be where one has the opportunity to finally design the House Made of Beauty—the house made of love and rainbow light, the house made of compassion and service, the house made of giving and getting the hearts desires, the house of knowledge, opportunity, and awareness, the house of good health, long life, and happiness.

Welcome home: hunter, farmer, and gatherer.
Welcome home scholar, musician, and artist.
Welcome home: mother, father, son, daughter, brother,
sister, aunt, uncle and cousin,
husband and wife.
Welcome home: scientist, carpenter, and oil field worker.
Welcome home: cook, jeweler, miner, and athlete.
Welcome home: all dogs, cats, and pets.
Welcome home: self.
Welcome home: all chickens and
egg gatherers and pig farmers, cow milkers,
and slaughterhouse workers.
Welcome home: all iPhone carriers and computer
workers sitting in darkened rooms.
Welcome home: the speakers of every tongue
and listeners of silent language.
Welcome: all religions, nationalities, and skin colors.
Welcome home: all those who went before,
making it possible for us to "be here now,"
thank you Ram Dass, and to those here now and to those
still in the ground and waiting to come.

Kiche migwech, thank you, Creator, thank you
very much, for all of the gifts.
Wewene, Kiche Migwech

(*Bodewadmi* [Potawatomi] language)

The Gratitude Principle resides with in our Sacred Flowering Tree center. Let us take some time now to breathe deeply. Centering, relocating, remembering, and repositioning ourselves as we trustingly, honorably, and confidently approach anew this great stream of life teachings in the manner and language upon which we have previously agreed, that of the Medicine Wheel

Teachings. At this time and place within our journey, let us now endeavor to move together in loose agreement and to be for a while "of one mind." Agreement on the use of this common language and symbol facilitates our inner/interactive dialogues about the Gratitude Principle and the sacred right of choice, and how this relates to ourselves and to the Medicine Wheel Path of Life. Consideration of this sacred medicine diagram, and our understanding and participation within it, constitute a metaphorical road map of knowledge that can, in time, create and maintain enhanced stability in our spiritual, mental, emotional, and physical realms.

THE GRATITUDE GIFTS AND OFFERINGS

Let us now assemble the honoring gifts once again, the high and personal inner gifts of qualities which only we can know, and the gifts of known and understood common tradition such as tobacco, water, or candles; chocolate, meats, fruits, or flowers; special drinks or nectars; ritual paintings, foods, cornmeal…and gifts of inspiration and the moment.

And come forward with these things in a spirit of unassuming and humble honoring.

Actually, we are the gift. Prepare to be taken…for our fealty is the sweetest payback and pay it forward that we can offer for the honor of being given the gift of life. This equation must be honored, lest the ledger grows unbalanced and little to big sacrifices are required to restore physical and spiritual balance:

Prayers over food are recognized—balancing, honoring, and grateful personal ceremonies.

> Notice, attention, and gratitude for "being breathed."
> Gratitude to the Father Sky-Sun for return at sunrise and sunset.
> Mindful Gratitude to the water beings as we drink, see, remember or feel them. Offeringsof cornmeal to the water beings are good.

Mindful Gratitude to the Fire Beings and an offering of liver is seen as good. Everything likes to eat, to see, and be clearly seen.

Speak in a friendly way to the Wind Beings…they know who we are and carry news everywhere!

Talk to a stone and a tree, a shrub, and the hill in the distance, "Hi, it's me, how ya' doin' today? You're pretty cute!"

Open the soles of your feet and invite them to "'pick up on" the Mother Earth as she vibrates and breathes through our bodies and connects with the upward solar rays of her lover. They are our elemental parents.

Go outdoors and lie first facedown, then turn to onto your back.

For the more adventurous, draw an arm's-length circle with a stick around you, think a little introductory offering of, "It's me here. Okay if I enter?" or, "I'm awful happy to have the time to do this." or, "I really don't know what I'm doing here," and sit there as unmoving as possible, except for the eyes, for at least twenty minutes or an hour. Some people like to pass the full time of a day and observe how it looks and feels. Notice and follow the breath until something else engages your attention. The natural world soon comes to accept our presence, and life picks up in ways we don't see when we are passing through at our natural pace. It is best if no food, water, or phone enters the circle or is in sight, smell, or earshot…and the sitting is best done in complete solitude. Try to brush off no bugs…they're on their way somewhere else. Then, when you are ready, stand up, or crawl out, noticing which direction you entered, faced, and departed. Try to make them the same. Then, make grateful farewells, and go. Remember the direction you faced in the mini-impromptu or temporary Medicine Wheel…it will reveal itself as important later. Smile.

Okay, I gotta go now…

March 18 at 20:53 CST

We really prefer to think of ourselves as immune to the very thought of any repercussions at all. Most of us originate out of a broad and pervasive cult of the individual, with a fairly complete sense of liberty of movement in place. Relative social and financial security has had a desensitizing effect on both cause and effect awarenesses and abundance has blunted sensory perceptions of the most subtle losses, thereby the causes and effects arising from balance and imbalance points in the natural world are downright scary, pooh-poohed, unregistered, or viewed as unimportant.

The Medicine Wheel Teachings present a natural and non-aligned "medicine way" by which we can rebuild or enhance sensitivity and gain a sense of oneself relative to values of the natural world that are held in common to everyone now alive on the Mother Earth.

We're all born at a certain time and that is our birth direction or season. Winter, spring, summer, or fall…what is yours? Prepare to enter it on the chart.

We all know what the time and season of this reading is. *Spring*…this knowing season marks the initial point of stepping onto the Medicine Wheel. That is home position two. Prepare to enter this on your chart. The time we first hear about and step onto the Medicine Wheel is the current passage of acquaintanceship, usually in a clockwise direction, from direction, or season to season. Occupying a "home" spot will likely be for a period of two-and-a-half years before moving on to another, not necessarily consecutive, direction. You may hear or read of this passage of time as "making a marriage" with this direction.

ART PROJECT

Draw an essential four-direction diagram of the Medicine Wheel with a center figure X dividing the seasons and a circle in the center denoting the home of the Sacred Flowering Tree, and then locate your "home" directions or gifts. The act of fitting personal facts upon and within this new presentation will begin to reorganize the pantheon of facts, personal timings, and placements in an original and totally noncompetitive way.

Optional color assignments and suggestions will follow in the next chapter.

March 19 at 20:53 CST

Color Vibrations, the Cradle and Web of Life

Visible color is a frequency of electromagnetic radiation. Color is a defined carrier and measurable source energy made visible, one that can pass through a vacuum. As we make an initial visit to the foundational Medicine Wheel–Gratitude diagram, intra/inter-twined, meshed and merged vibrant and creative systems that are designed to lend understanding, credibility, visibility, and a measure of valuable objectivity to the intense subjectivity of narrow and contracted individual histories, truths, memories, and focus. Still, this is the diagrammatic format and the color data that is immediately seen to be forthcoming from the identified "home" directions, which will attract and anchor attention. Before even observing additional personal data more closely, let us begin to further open and initiate sensory and some additional perceptions, and permit them to consider functioning in the broadened fields of the Medicine Wheel basics. There is no need, or desirability at this point, to analyze, quantify, or qualify any of the data. Let us simply relax the fact-finding and processing reflexes and allow attention and awareness to relax and soak in the initial Medicine Wheel diagram, its directional attributes and the colors of this "Cradle" and Web of Life, as the colors effectively "wrap around" the optical spectrum as a closed loop. Study on these things: Soon your personal choice points and experience will reveal additional affinities, and entries will follow.

Direction	Color	Season	Attribute	Quality
East—Sun	Yellow	Spring	Mental	Illumination, inspiration
South—Earth	Red	Summer	Heart	Trust, innocence
West—Water	Black	Fall	Physical	Medicine, mystery
North—Air	White	Winter	Spirit	Wisdom, being breathed
Center	Blue	Wholeness	Wholeness	Wholeness

The up above, the down below, and the all around are also qualities and directions, as are the connecting linear and circular life paths that serve to link and connect all applied and collected aspects of an Earth walk.

The Center, where the Sacred Flowering Tree stands rooted, is connected and incorporated into each of the seasons and is the enduring center-cross point where directional paths cross the center when passing from one direction to another, instead of progressing around the circle in a clockwise way. But, principally, the Center represents a locus point of spirit origin and return after all of the directional paths have been "walked" and the directional *home* "marriages" are made.

So with the paths and identifying marks of the Earth walk, we hunt for ourselves, tracking ourselves through the sparkling winter snows, blowing frosty breaths, through "the quiet time of listening," attuning our senses with the chosen seeds and the still somnolent Mother Earth...connecting with this year's dream of life; on through the summer work of making flower, fruit, and new seed production; to the autumn work of completion and harvest; culminating in the return ceremonies of "firing the summer-made seeds of inspiration" for the new year.

The inspiration of this spring vision begins earlier, in the storytelling time of the White Winter plain of winter. The year originates in winter, travels from winter to spring, then summer to autumn, only to make the return to the year's origin: winter. The heavy lifting of return, the reception, the selection and firing of seeds; prayer, celebration, and rest of winter prepares the way for the dream of life to be enriched with our northern, white Spirit of Winter genius and heart. Here and now we fertilize and merge with the seed sacs of eternity to link our walks and destinies with the heartbeat of the awakening Mother Earth as she stirs to receive fecund shafts of fire.

Somewhere around the Spring Equinox, our yellow Mind of Spring seed sacs are joined, warmed and enlightened by the strengthening and balancing Creative fires of our Father Sky-Sun, as he reaches for the Mother to initiate the spring marriage talks. The red summer heart of trust is emboldened to flourish, making new year's seed from fruit, vegetable, and nut; the black medicine face of autumn receives the golden east light through the turning leaves. Here is an east to west medicine crossing... we see more clearly how the Medicine Wheel gradually demonstrates its truths to us and how the natural world lives by its laws. This line moves from the east, the mental plane, and crosses the center and connects with the west, the physical plane. This path is called the "hard road of life" because it spans the mind-east (mental) and physical-west (body) axis.

Drawing the year to a close, the seasons complete themselves and return to their seat in the northern, white wisdom, Winter medicine. Here, the connection of south, red heart and trust medicine, crosses the center and connects with the white wisdom, Winter medicine. This passage is called "the Good Red Road," because it connects the sympathetic elements of the trusting heart with that of spiritual wisdom. All of our paths must, can, and will be walked. None are to be denied—postponed perhaps, but not denied permanently. Our center can only be fully arrived at and resided in when we arrive with the full complement of the life/directional experiences we have earned, experiences derived and honed through the directional walks and visits. The center is a well-known place where an aspect of us always lives, because it is an origination point only fully and completely arrived at when all of the paths have been walked and the marriages made. One can reasonably expect to make several circumambulations of the wheel in a given lifetime or Earth walk, so, no hurry.

To accomplish these circle walks, conscious time will be spent in each direction where the experiences and influences will offer and contribute all of the valuable life skills necessary with which to build and stock the shelving of our inner storehouses with love, wisdom, and knowledge, trust, inspiration and illumination, mystery, courage and endurance; all within a self-crafted cradle and rainbow web of life designed to support our newness, the essential framework, understandings, direction, gifts, and spirit of the Medicine Wheel Teachings and the Gratitude Principle: knowledge, balance and harmony…all ways…all days…now and forever more…*Ehe*, yes!

This is one trustworthy Way among many by which to view the infinity of our personal subjective perspective as it interfaces within the well-known and understood framework of Creative objectivity, as we know it. The gifts of the Mother and the Father, our elemental parents are and continue to be the first, most beautiful and enduring of gifts, barring our being breathed alive, that the Creator, the Master of All Breath, gave to us. May all blessings be upon us as we live and are breathed alive within this miracle of Creation. May our centered and deepest selves always know joy and happiness.

SPIRIT TALK

Welcome home traveler, seeker, and seer. And so, by these ways may we seek, find, understand, and truly see not only ourselves but all others, as well.

March 14, 2014, 23:14:59 CST

The Book of Earth Days…Grounding Beauty, Part 1

Grounding Beauty

In the last days of the "white plain" of late, late winter and early, early spring, in the days of seeming nothingness, remain alert and maintain awareness of your first feelings. Everything is present in spirit, thought, and intent before the first toe wiggles or leaves a track upon the skin of our Mother. Everything—even us.

Like a tracker hunting a snowshoe rabbit, its white hair lost to the hunter's eye in late sparkling snow, the rabbit cannot be entirely seen but it has left a sign of progress—a passing track. So also can we now view ourselves as each element; tracking our progress, temporarily invisible even to ourselves in the White Plain of spiritual evolution just prior to the spring emergence, but leaving a discernable passing track. We *are* able to measure our progress.

Like a hungry fox, forced from the den by a growling stomach and perhaps a litter of nursing kits, she emerges to sniff the air and then, her lucky moment—she picks up rabbit smell. Bounding off, then stealthily picking up her feet high, she begins creeping forward low on her belly until it is time to leap fast and, hopefully, land right on top of the snowshoe before it can do more than roll a panicked eye and initiate a frenzied leap. Too late…

Like the tracker, like the fox, we are all hunters and trackers of our happiness. In order to successfully realize, fulfill, and satisfy the hunt, let us identify and name just a few of the many gifts, situations, and conditions that may come to occupy space in the circle of our consciousness, or unconsciousness, by which to power and employ our objectives: our strengths and hungers; cunnings, camouflages, and negotiations; feints and attacks; persuasions, lures, and traps; patience and charm; promises of reward or loss; surrenders, treaties, bargains, and contracts—an awesome arsenal certainly. But prior to employing these rudimentary secondary tools, the hunter of happiness and satisfaction must sniff for the invisible signs of the prey. Yet the quarry may not solely be intended for food, mating, or survival. The quarry may be the raw material of evolution and understating, as we, the hunter and the quarry, are always in a coexistent and mutable relationship with one another.

Of no less import are the quarries of happiness, of interactive appreciation and recognition of growth and beauty, calm and peace—building, farming, nurturing, and creating. These tracks and scents are also present, and more subtly so, than the survival skills. But many of the earlier signals emerging out of the white plain will herald prescience, a "knowingness" of these things… things still hidden or invisible for the moment, for the moment…

Specialized hunting and recognition skills can be taught, observed, developed, honed, and refined in order to recognize the *approach* of these energetic signals of emergence and revelation, and those of actual physical approaches and presences. Skills of appreciation and the memory and knowledge of previous seasons are the snares by which the more esoteric beauties may be captured and grounded. These skills must be kept as close as a breeze, fog, or mist in order to register and evaluate emergences of Spirit in the moments just prior to its showing a physical face.

And this memory and knowledge is built, stored, revealed, accessed, and released from within and upon the Medicine Wheel of Life.

March 15 at 12:29 CST

And so, the natural world, the Mother Earth, the Father Sky-Sun and all emergent life forms are fully moment to moment, downloading, releasing, and broadcasting new life codes and information designed to inculcate and elucidate all sentient and non-sentient beings with energetic messages of the past, present, and the new season. However, one should be appraised and prepared in advance to understand that the initial willingness to examine, comprehend, and handle these broadcasts requires a renewed commitment to our previously seated, and new, diligent practices of sharpened awarenesses, accompanied by the willingness of our deepest inner spirit to meet, seat, and integrate coherent, and perhaps previously unknown or forgotten, tools of comprehension for the growth of a potentially expanded present and future intelligence. Be it also posted that certain habits, histories, and positions will probably be called up for review, purification, renewal, retooling, or dismissal and necessarily examined for their current status regarding inherent reliability and desirability factors.

The little red schoolhouse of "original instruction" is both thorough and deep. Enter here only the stout and loving of heart. As an aspirant or provisional scholar of the original instructions, open your eyes even wider, look deep and long to the natural world as a prime mentor of the first degree—first among many principal mentors and systems relating to a successful life experience upon and within this beautiful Mother Earth and Father-Sky Sun, our spot of divinely radiant Creation.

This platform, no matter what our background or training, is what we have. And this platform, which cannot be stressed or emphasized enough, is everything. All wisdom and knowledge is to be found in the natural world—mathematics, vibration, sound, color and light, speech, thought, emotion, and movement. The experience of a unified self in real connection with every other living thing is within the reach and possibility of us all, through the process of developing and accepting enhanced sensitivity to the natural world.

The deepest and most ephemeral tools of diaphanous and delicate information-gathering are designed to promulgate fuller life experiences. These are tools of creative fiber, prehensile information gathering tools, which may appear or be experienced as feelings or presentiments. They are innate tools that may be intuited and absorbed from life-carrying water droplets within the fogs, mists, snows, or rains, which are taken deep within our bodies through breath, drink, or skin sensations. Tools and message bearers are constantly being beamed from the great central Sun and the related Fire Beings; the tendrils of new smoke voices support and energize all of our inner fire–driven and physical activities. Tools and message bearers of refined planetary movers like the winds, which carry spirits and information to the Spirit and material world, and the tools of the animal and plant kingdoms, which carry food, information, and deep nourishment in the form of physical food, wake-up bird song, our song, and last but not least, the ever-present emergent Mother vibrations and new spirit voices that are communicated through the feet, mind, and skin, Spirit, prayer, and emotion.

This is the deepest "medicine" preparation for the new cycle— spring. This platform, or dance, is also present in other forms, but similar in nature, at the closure and advent of all other seasons, the seasons of the natural world and those of the male and female two-leggeds of Spirit incarnate, the human beings. We must be taught how to be fully human. The original instructions can be pointed out to us by other human teachers whose eyes are wider open than ours, or we can open our own eyes wider in order to see, feel, and come to know these original instructions for ourselves. And the teachings are self-evident and ever present in the natural world.

Spring is the opening "good medicine" and primal pattern of our world of duality. Here we prepare to take our place within the grand and mysterious scheme of creation by tilling the inner fields and cultivating both the inner and outer gardens of ongoing life. Come, let us take up the rakes, pruning shears, and hoes forged of willingness, acceptance, flexibility, and gratitude to become the diligent, enthusiastic, and energetic farmers of our lives that we, deep in our hearts, know ourselves to be. This season initiates all personal and collective ceremonies and is the father, mother, and child of all other ceremonies. As this season goes by, remain attentive to the gains assessed and chosen, or not chosen, to be brought forward as your personal "medicine"—driven, revealed, shared, or gifted by this hard won intelligence. Take these things unto yourself for your consideration; live, sing, dance, pray, and grow by them. Share and giveaway as much as is appropriate, timely, and possible; synthesize, add to, delete, test, and build the edifice of grounded beauty as only one person, ourselves, can... and become our own precious seed, sprout, flower, fruit, nut, and bare root again as only we can. *Aho!*

We are always becoming. It is good. It is very, very good. And so, we are readied for this and all future seasons, no matter what they may bring and how they might appear, so we may never, ever, forget that we *are* "the sacred."

March 15 at 12:38 CST

SPIRIT TALK

Grounding Beauty

And now, the south winds pick up, the thunder beings speak and the rains begin. *Aho!*

They have spoken.

March 15, 2014, 17:54:30 CST

Merging With Beauty, For Our Ears Only

We have followed our heads as long as possible. Oh, we love our heads *so* much, yet the head only knows, but feelings that merge with happiness can only fully happen within the heart. Mind can come along, but only, along. The mind cannot be permitted to remain in ascendancy. It must be coaxed, friended, tricked, reasoned, or habituated into some semblance of partnership with the heart, for the mind *knows* so beautifully, yet it cannot feel emotion. Shock, yes, and chemically and hormonally stimulated energetic surges, yes, and the mind becomes much smarter, more valuable, and trustworthy when functioning as a part of the whole mind, heart, body construct toward the ultimate goal of a unified consciousness.

To merge with beauty and happiness is to connect, to flow into and within a personally located core energy. What is that? For the time being, let us allow the sacred diagram of the Medicine Wheel and of the Sacred Flowering Tree to represent a shared visual and common language/symbol with the Circle, representing the all and ever present Spirit, and view ourselves as *being* within the center, the Tree of Life, grounding earthly beauty and aspirating the solar manna that powers system and movement. Yes. Let the branches reach. No mind. Tree. Simple and complete unity, beingness…

The tree cannot move, but exercises knowingness and beingness within the core energy, freely circulating and available to those known mostly in the dream or vision stage; the station of the waiting soul and embryo; the more precipitate stages of life forms coming closer to linking with physical form and energy; those beings now emerging from the pendulous amniotic spirit sacs of light and unity, approaching the force fields of gravity, vision, form, and, *aah*, the duality—the big game, the main event on the horizon in this galaxy, as far as we know.

Paths we have all walked to arrive at this place, the now, the eternal present, are the paths we traveled while still without form. Paths that are largely forgotten but for spirit escapes into the dream or the creative void, but no less real, viable, and laden with a treasure trove of sentient and emotional personal histories of the most plastic and mind-bending qualities. Our story. Everyone and every being's story and personal path is one of hunting happiness and grounding beauty. The huntress, the hunter, and the quarry must include the full landscape of preform and physical-form spirit treks and journeys; surfing the extreme light and dark waves of the midday and the midnight, illuminated now by shooting star, north and pole star, now morning star, then evening star; full moons, blood moons, darks of the moon; eclipses, solstices, equinoxes of sun, solar flare, and wind; spirit helpers, guardians, guides, angels, animal helpers, observers, ones we should give a wide berth and keep moving; creative voids; unknown lands, sight, people, colors, smell, texture, and messages. Messages deeply encoded within us and originating from core source must be recovered to reconstitute the missing parts that bear seminal stories of how we came to be and serve to lend courage, endurance, and bravery to the naked walk of the hairless and defenseless two-legged, making the lonely walk of often veiled and obfuscated consciousness.

But, hang on…we hold the cards of core energetic star origin, yes. And we hold the cards of the original gifts, the physical creations of form within the duality principle that we honor and call by the names: *Our Mother, the Earth, and our Father, the Sky-Sun, as the first, most beautiful and enduring gifts of the prime Creator, the Master of All Breath.*

Yes, and now our precious forms. We have gotten out, survived, and succeeded by the skin of our teeth time and again. Now, it is our personal journey and sacred charge to put together all of the pieces again, yes, and again hunt beauty and happiness. Walk all the paths of the Medicine Wheel without shame, blame, or guilt, gaining lost, stolen, and forgotten pieces of divinity, light, and humanity. Yes, to again hunt beauty and happiness by walking all the beauty paths and calling or making the names, songs, and dances of life with recognition, laughter, tears, and breaking sobs of joy and heartbreak. (Oh, God, I'm breaking into a sweat while writing this and have to take off a sweater and socks. If this old gal can do it, you can.) Go! Do! Be! It is said that the Creator loves our blood, sweat, and tears. Don't hold back. Hunt your happiness in yourself and merge with beauty, love, and wisdom, then it will be found everywhere and in all living things.

Personal ceremonies of communication, language, and liberty are the lifeblood of our existence.

March 16 at 8:16 CST

Communication, Language, and Liberty

There is also the language of Spirit, and of the body, but here we will examine the predominately silent and insistent voices of Spirit. As autonomous beings, we are tasked with the very interesting job of recognizing that each of us possesses an inner language as unique as our fingerprint, DNA, and blood makeup; as unique as history writ within a rainbow scale of skin or strand of hair. The language of Spirit is a second city or village within which we coexist. We knowingly, or unknowingly, call it intuition, now a hunch, now second sight, now a lie. We may call it stupid, say "Where's your proof?" We may think it is questionable, or perhaps the worst denial occurs when a human miscreant is seen or heard casting the ultimate character aspersion by identifying information arising from the language of Spirit as (shudder) "dark, or lost witchcraft.." This person is either a serious troublemaker, in command of a serious truth, or seriously out of touch with the more complexly layered or unknown realities of an unknown language spoken or demonstrated by another.

The tasking of our diligent attention becomes so much richer and interesting when viewed in this manner. *Hmm*…additional languages to think about. We all know that occasionally our voices, words, thought forms, actions, and eyes belie our reality or truth…*Hmm,* there, the receding water is revealing the gasping mollusks, saw grasses, and bacterial life of inner language, experiencing an evolutionary emergency. This is one obvious time and place to begin looking deeply, through the clearing throat or sweaty palms, at this discrepancy before it gets hidden by socially accepted white lies, courtesy forms, the exigencies of work, or salving the feelings of others. And then, the deepest cut comes when the language and the information contained within it becomes so successfully managed that the entity no longer knows of it and is troubled no more. It will often be called: denial, out of touch, unconscious; slow, touched, and when the communication membrane thickens further, perhaps, autistic or in some other manner distorted or shifted.

March 16 at 9:57 CST

Do not be afraid of or shrink from observing intently and testing the findings that emerge out of Spirit language contact and the surrounding fields. The very real possibility of errors in perception or interpretation will exist, as it interfaces with the filters of the emotional and desire body of the heart and the logical construct of the mental plane. We must be as ready and willing to admit mistakes or question ourselves, as we are to question others, and we must be willing to admit our mistakes and initiate correction. The true messages of the Spirit language can withstand questions from any direction, and when attention develops into a true habitual scan and response reflex, then trust in our processes will grow. When one is fully or even partially attuned to the personal Spirit language, it becomes exciting and interesting. Our world becomes first larger, and then potentially all encompassing. Then another very interesting thing occurs.

As energy and attention broadens upon the wheel, proportionally more energy is allocated away from previous limited principal areas of the emotional heart and mental planes, as informational gathering and experiential platforms expand. As our attention broadens in a trusted and radiant format, more information and experiential opportunities are available, and beautifully attractive. So, happiness has been hunted and beauty grounded. A visit has been made and we are more confident that the findings represent truth. Trust that the time and energy spent here will go "into the till," so to speak, of larger life experience and other nonnegotiable shouldered responsibilities and duties.

Be aware that all processes may now begin to function more smoothly and enjoyably. They will be uniquely yours. Less energy and directed thought will be expended, and the "white plain" of the northern Spirit Mind will enter, seat, and make its contribution of a more calm and effortless knowing. Thinking still happens. Affairs of life, love, and desires of the heart still happen. The body still happens. Now, balanced spirit increasingly happens. No one system is in the permanent ascendancy and, as a direct side effect, each system benefits from not always having to "be the one" or being forced to carry a disproportionate load of operational responsibility. Be prepared for these shifts by simply allocating less importance to keeping the mind always busy and occupied. It can happen. You can afford a little time off to do this. Actually, this is a completely private and personal decision and, as such, will possibly not even be perceived by others as happening, assuming you are not at an office desk. Carve out a little time, at least as much time as you spend brushing your teeth. [Smiles.] Okay, now let's assume that you've found a little personal time for an exploratory practice. Prepare to allow some openness into the brain and relax into "being" through aware choice, "be breathed," participate in regular sunrise and sunset greetings, meditation, exercise, yoga, love, right livelihood and service, and some kind of a daily practice of prayer or ceremony.

Find and design your own meaningful ceremonies. Take a class, go on a camping trip, tie a few flies, call on someone who needs some attention that you just "haven't found the time" to call on, volunteer, catch up on sleep, clip and file your finger and toenails, trim bristling nose hairs, purchase one good food and eliminate one food not so good for yourself, listen to or make some music; sing, dance, or write; show the child, husband or wife, parent, friend, dog, plant, or house or office that you really care by the quality of attention that can arise out of a mind that is not overly filled with whatevers. Dust, for heaven's sake and really feel the action and really listen to and hear the medicine sound a broom makes as it whisks, whisks, whisks its way across the floor. Mind where you live! Put down the phone! Don't take it *everywhere*! It takes up our emotional and mental attention to the point that we live in a constant "on point" position, a state of being available to who knows what. Well, how about turning it off, putting it down occasionally and, *gasp*, being solitarily available to ourselves?

Until our inner languages of mind, heart, body, and spirit are integrated and balanced, we will not be able penetrate or untangle the mixed language messages of others. How often is the question raised? What does he/she really mean? We must quiet our inner language congestion to find understanding!

As in any communication and spoken, thought, or written language, intent and listening skills must continually be examined, so that meaning and intent remain in fine attunement, harmony, and balance, calling for the most appropriate evaluation with the compassion and consideration needed to honor and satisfy the feelings and needs of ourselves and others. An assessment, as accurate as possible, of just how much and what degree of information is called for must always be a part of every conversation, be it spoken, written word, or thought form.

It is no wonder that so much knowledge and wisdom has been lost, discredited (sometimes by ourselves), maligned, jeered at and just simply not "gotten" or understood. Simultaneously, a certain depth and richness of spiritual understanding and practice recedes like water in a tide pool when the going gets too tough. The more complex nuances of spoken and unspoken communication contract, receding as dropping waterlines, while nourishing tidal flows disappear into the distance. Life changes in the now dry or muddy flats. Survival and adaption steps up, perfectly producing life forms that can live, producing what? New languages. So, adaptation still calls for attention, awareness, and consciousness shifts of every sort in order for us to comprehend more than personal new inner and outer landscapes, but also those of every other.

Going deeper…we must do our best to be the vigilant hunter of visiting thought forms. Some passing thoughts we can own, some we cannot, and of those, we had better run down and identify the point of origin lest they take up undocumented residences, come to masquerade as ourselves and braid into our consciousness, language, and even intent, erroneously or, at most, innocuously, ignorantly. It is at this moment, and not a moment later, that it becomes of paramount importance to discriminate, choose, and identify by what means we will allow ourselves to be educated, manipulated, or influenced, and the converse. It is always the time to smarten up and pay attention to every little thing. It is always, and ever, up to us, at least since we have chosen to reside within this, the ultimate choice platform of duality and the springboard of unity.

It is from the unified and receptive language interaction of our mind, heat, body, and spirit languages that we are able to communicate with the realities and even messages from denizens of the natural world—refreshing and newly emerging spirit beings in the forms of plants, animals, the Grandmother Moon and Star Beings, the Wind, Fire, and Water Beings, and even the heartbeat of Mother Earth, the pulses of the Father Sky-Sun, and the mind of the Prime Creator, the Master of All Breath. Now *that* is communication. Let's go!

March 16 at 8:23 CST

If all base languages possess their own unique and original qualities, they also possess qualities in common with other, probably not all, vibrational frequencies. Therefore, if we are not "'different'"…are we the same?

Languaging, Hunting Happiness, and Grounding Beauty, Working Together

The Medicine Wheel 4 x 4 wagon is building its wheels. The finely meshed and recognized gears of language that can carry our loads, provide a center and direction, are beginning to be directionally and seasonally purposed to function as an inclusive true home and spiritual sanctuary. The home is under final construction and livable…always a dance and a song in the process of *becoming* at spring, or *any* given time.

Welcome home traveler and seeker.

March 15 at 18:18 CST

SPIRIT TALK

The quality of mind, heart, thought, word, and intention, as well as service and action, remain the most important considerations signifying successful "hunts for happiness" and "grounding beauty" activities. It is here that personal medicine is built and comes together within an initiated and sacred Earth walk of mindful, fresh and ever-changing ceremony.

SPRING EQUINOX

March 21

The east-west arm of balance is the "hard road of life." The east-west axis provides the essential cross balance with the north-south cross balance–spinal axis of harmony—the "Good Red Road," road of the marriage of the southern heart and northern seat of purity and wisdom.

This mental spring arm extends forward and out from the center, joining with the introspective, medicine autumn arm of the autumnal equinox.

The Medicine Wheel is in an active and visible building process.

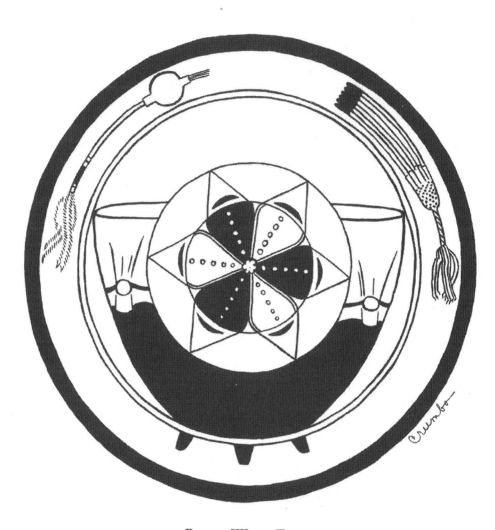

Peyote Water Drum

*The Peyote Water Drum of the Native American Church rests within its
Sun and Moon, and speaks of the collective voice of Mankind raised
in a prayer of gratitude and thanks to the Creator.*

Peyote Water Drum
Minisa Crumbo

Cultivation of the Divine Inner Garden

Gratitude Principle Teaching, Day 1

BozHo nikan—hello, my bone,

And now, let us think on the myriad of things that have been placed into motion through loving and energetic intention in order that our world might go on "in a good way."

Our visit about the previous sets of twenty-one days has now brought us to the mindful celebration of all that has gone into the planning the new year. This brings us to a moment of release, trust, gratitude, and into a spirit of willing integration with the fullness of Creation as manifested by the seasonal markers of continuance and reemergence into the new. Now is a time that we might study on core meaningful alliances, those personal and those collective. May we consent and give ourselves a well-deserved opportunity to surrender and to view, remember and experience ourselves as aspects of and parts of the larger whole of this unfolding with and into the natural world. That we may breathe and be breathed as our holy and sacred hearts, minds, bodies, and spirits *are*, cogent and integral, within the emergent vision of yet another season, as we bravely extend new shoots, buds, blooms, and unfurled leaf potential as manifested through our dreams, hope, words, prayers, and activities.

SPIRIT TALK

As we do the next right things that appear before us, let us pray that each and every one of us move sweetly and with gratitude within the delicate mists of Creation, floating within each of our personal emergent myths, as precious elements of a renewed cycle within yet another emerging myth of the great mystery.

A blessing is bestowed upon us yet again.

Aho! It is good. It is very, very good.
Migwech, wewene kiche migwech.

—Dawn Woman

Gratitude Principle Teaching, Day 2

Thursday, April 5, 2012

BozHo nikan—hello, my bone,

The twenty-one-day cultivation of the spring divine garden may be approached by electing to revisit our golden heart center and identifying it as the *first* and *elemental* Garden of Eden. A good place to *begin*, considering that this looking is done by gazing out of the window with the intention of remembering and renewing our relationship with the natural world. The natural world is a proven and worthy gift, indeed the first, most enduring and beautiful gift from the Creator, and thereby also the most trusted tool with which to ally our core values of unconditional love and divine potential. Remember to breathe and be breathed, as we reform natural alliances with our inner garden. Allow or envision the inner garden to be grounded in the golden and loving light of the Father Sky-Sun and the rootedness of the unconditional love of the Mother Earth. This is the essential inner garden from which all else will emerge. In spirit or physically, make some tobacco ties and hang them around the dedicated inner or outer space. Bless it and ask for it to be an integral part of the annual blessing of *all* fields and beasts of the fields, the inner and outer fields of Creation. We cultivate the inner fields first through reception and willingness, remembering, always, that we are inseparable aspects of all that is sacred and divine.

Play, divinely play, with small and reasonable possibilities, for instance, playfully and gratefully examine any sweetgrass shoots, listen to spring bird calls, water the house plants, dust or clean out some small drawer or shelf, look or step outside and notice the mists, winds, and clouds, get plenty of sleep and a good soup in you. Open a fresh pack of crackers to go with it. Call someone who needs to hear from you, journal, visit someone who cannot get out, look deep into pet eyes and the eyes of two-legged loved ones. Send love, without expecting return, to known and unknown places that need heart nourishing and encouragement. Turn over some ground with the golden plow of love. When the energetic sky has been set and some ground has been plowed, select some personal vegetable or flower seeds, such as bachelor buttons, peas, lettuce, something light, colorful and personally simple and pleasing, and symbolically plant them. And then, forget that you are within the twenty-one-day time. That has been done and will take its own course. Very importantly, as a daily and moment-to-moment activity, endeavor to express gratitude for *everything*—experienced, heard about, or even thought of—even if you cannot fully feel it yet. In this way, we supply the fertilizer and water for the building of core gratitude by remembering to reflect *all* to the backboard of the golden light of loving Creation, thereby building, building, building our store of positive automatic responses, which will be available to come forward and offer aid in times of stress, inquiry, or need. Even if we cannot approve of or accept certain things, we can at least give them permission to *be,* and therefore move somewhat out of the undesirable quarter of judgment, and from that endurance, bravery, patience, will come *inspiration, illumination*—the essential qualities of spring can and will emerge.

SPIRIT TALK

You, your circle, family, and tribe are doing the final inner work of preparing the energetic and physical circle into which the beloved will enter and find a place of trust and love prepared for them.

—Dawn Woman
Posted at 4:29 CST

Friday, April 6, 2012

Gratitude Principle Teaching, Day 3

BozHo nikan—hello, my bone,
   Look upon the robes of the Mother Earth and invite a color(s) to walk with you.

—Dawn Woman

Reflections: I take off my shoes and walk barefoot on the Mother Earth, today.

I…_____

_____

_____

_____

_____

_____

_____

_____

_____

_____

_____

_____

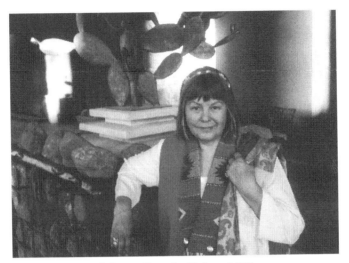

Minisa Crumbo Halsey, 2011

Gratitude Principle Teaching, Day 4

BozHo nikan—hello, my bone,

It's "Redbud Winter" in the heartland of America, Sweet Medicine land, and magenta is a special color for now. Today, we will seek the Father Sky-Sun, whether it is shining or behind clouds, state our name, and invite him into our "grateful place" where our current spirit colors already reside. We allow the Father Sky-Sun to illuminate, vitiate, warm, and saturate our color...soak in it...breathe it...be it...to do something original, revolutionary, or outrageous with it and not to tell anyone...or tell everyone.

Redbud winter–Dawn Woman
Posted at 7:00 CST

Color is the frequency of a vibration.

Reflections on my favorite seasonal colors:

_____

_____

_____

_____

_____

_____

_____

_____

_____

_____

Sunday, April 8, 2012

Gratitude Principle Teaching, Day 5

BozHo nikan—hello, my bone,

Practice a mindful and grateful walk and sleep upon the Mother Earth.

—Dawn Woman
Posted at 5:17 CST

Sleep is a Spirit Walk.

Reflections on sleeping and walking:

_____

_____

_____

_____

_____

_____

_____

_____

_____

_____

_____

_____

_____

_____

_____

_____

_____

_____

_____

Monday, April 9, 2012

Gratitude Principle Teaching, Day 6
The Spring Ceremony

BozHo nikan—hello, my bone,

This day we will consider visiting the natural world of the Mother Earth and the Father Sky-Sun as a child. We two-leggeds are walking erect color-beings of the season, capable of recognizing and celebrating ourselves as children of our divine Mother Earth and Father Sky-Sun's, our natural parents, union, and in doing so we may remember ourselves and all others, as direct physical issue of their loving relationship.

In the old honoring language...it is good to make an honoring prayer from the "grateful place." Spit or blow into an offering of tobacco four times, and then "put down" the gift of the tobacco being, Se'-Ma', onto the Mother Earth. Now, offer honoring tobacco to the Father Sky-Sun in the same way. The order of offering may differ, just observe and view yourself as being Spirit guided.

Take a snapshot of yourself...any way...and see what comes forward. Just you, as you are to yourself.

WE ARE ALWAYS BECOMING

Tomorrow is the seventh day of the twenty-one days we have set aside to ask for and to prepare for the new season and the new endeavors, both those named and those unnamed.

And now, we will prepare to mark, honor, and celebrate this segment of consecrated time with a feast or a fast. You may begin thinking of that and preparing at this time. Either way, if it rains or snows, consider collecting some of the "new water," dip a finger into it and touch the top of your head four times, as the personal unification Water Beings blessing, and then drink some, slowly,

slowly, slowly. If it does not rain or snow, honor what water is available to you. You may know of some caught clean water outside that you may work with. If there is enough water, many things may be done with it, like ritually bathing the head, hair, face, body, eyes, wrists, and using it for cooking, plants...

If the wild green onions are up, make a tobacco offering from the grateful place: say your name and ask permission, and then you may take up a sharp stone for cutting or use your fingernail for gathering. Use no metal. Both the top and root bulb may be cleaned and eaten. You will then have some first harvest onions for a steamed wild onion meal with scrambled eggs, and tofu or hamburger. If no wild onions are available to you, select a fresh green of your choice from the store.

THE FIRST FOOD OF THE SEASON

The wild onions can be one of the first honoring feasts of the season. And in so doing, it will be recognized as a direct giveaway from the natural world to ourselves and the other greens eaters towards the strong maintenance of physical life. The wild onions giveaway of their lives is intended to purify and thin our blood for the coming season.

SPIRIT TALK

And so, with these ways and many others, we reconnect and renew to our Earth walks...in balance and harmony with all sentient and non-sentient beings and observing our new myths as they evolve, unfold, and reveal themselves woven by our *breaths* into the warp and woof of our livesand *all* other lives.

Aho!

Bama mine, See you later,
Dawn Woman
Posted 5:42 CST

Gratitude Principle Teaching, Day 7

Tuesday, April 10, 2012

BozHo nikan—hello my bone,

This day we stand within the sacred seven.

And now, as a serious progression deeper into the Gratitude Principle Teachings, we begin to express gratitude for *each* and *every* thing present in our lives, even those things for which we might not actually be grateful. Speak these words to yourself, "I am glad that 'thus and so,' is this way," naming the present issue in mind.

Do not be surprised if your response is a mixed one of fear, sorrow, wild laughter, or anger and *not* gratitude. You are now moving into the core dynamic of the Gratitude Principle. It is designed to *bring up* certain things (history) that can begin moving into your Center and be stationed for *dynamic change* and *departure* from your mind, heart, and bodily (cellular) history. It may take a while to discharge certain issues (history, thought forms, or memories) but trust that each subsequent time these things *voluntarily* arise in response to you saying, "I am glad," that you are not making new trouble for yourself or revisiting fruitless old issues, but that your inner pump is priming and bringing up the old issues for release. It may take quite a few visits to the said issue for this to be accomplished, perhaps quite a while.

Remember and *trust* that you are residing for the time being in Sacred Ceremony in order to live life in a good way. This is a hard Way but a good Way…it is a reliable way to internally *purify* and *renew* while at the same time setting yet another of the trusted pools of automatic responses of *gratitude* and positive, loving reservoirs in place. These actions are building automatic responses by which to live.

If some history or circumstance is just too difficult to go deeply into, do not do so.

CHOICE IS A SACRED RIGHT—MINE AND YOURS

You may not feel well from time to time, or feel that you look good (but *remember* you are in Ceremony!). This is to be expected. It is also to be expected that you may regret having embarked upon this ceremony, so, soften up on yourself and try to keep going, if you can at all. Others, with "Spirit Eyes" *will see* you and know that you are doing a sacred thing. They will look upon you with love and perhaps smile. Do not be surprised. It will validate your experience and serve to make you feel very, very good.

SPIRIT TALK

At the conclusion of the twenty-one days, much will have been created, discovered, and resolved, but for now, we are at the second threshold of deepening the Grateful Place by practice. Each day and movement takes us deeper into the loving mind with which the Creator designed, created, and continues to create our world. Let us *remember* ourselves as sparks of the divine and continue to take up the sacred labor and charge of becoming *co-creators* of our lives and keeping the world alive by our labor and prayer.

Bama mine, See you later,
Dawn Woman

Wednesday, April 11, 2012

Gratitude Principle Teaching, Day 8

BozHo nikan,

Breathe, release, and integrate…

Bama mine,
Dawn Woman

Reflections on "being breathed":

_____

_____

_____

_____

_____

_____

_____

_____

_____

_____

Thursday, April 12, 2012

Gratitude Principle Teaching, Day 9

BozHo Nikan,

From the Grateful Place, this is a good day to review, sift through, and renew stated and as yet unformed intention.

Bama mine,
Dawn Woman
Posted at 5:20 CST

Reflections and review:

_____

_____

_____

_____

_____

_____

_____

_____

_____

_____

Friday, April 13, 2012

Gratitude Principle Teaching, Day 10

BozHo nikan,

Today, locate the Grateful Place and penetrate it with all of your externalized intention, fertilizing the humming nucleus of every cell and thereby shifting your vision into a position of dynamic change and radiance.

Activation…

Bama mine,
Dawn Woman
Posted at 24:02 CST

Reflections on things for which I am grateful:

_____

_____

_____

_____

_____

_____

_____

_____

Gratitude Principle Teaching, Day 11

Saturday, April 14, 2012

BozHo nikan—Greetings,

UNIFY

This day, allow yourself all the time you feel you need in order to mindfully greet and graciously receive the newly conceived and perceived intentions and those proven and worthy alliances, aspirations, and eternal connections with Divine Origin.

This day, revisit the new ground of your personal inner season and that of our shared outer season of the natural world—worlds now rife with potential and resplendently attired in the shiny news of emergence. For as these things have emerged into the present moment, know that they have freshly crept from the warm and humming nucleus of the Mother Earth and Father Sky-Sun's active conversation, a conversation of *unity*, much like our own inner conversations of humming center and highest intention, producing the purifying and energizing power to support, encourage, and drive the new.

UNITY

This day, allow yourself *all* of the time you feel you need to survey, acquaint, and sort through your inner landscape that is sister and brother mirror to the *all* of Creation.

There remains the ongoing labor of processing history that is worthy of rejoining the great energy field through the mutual release consent mechanism of the Gratitude Principle. These labors run alongside of, but are not separate from, the concurrent creative unity practices and observances. Endeavor to have some fun and erudition with both and all fields of divine play…

Play in the inner fields of the divine and gather the intention of incipient emergence energy. Make ready and give permission for those things (charged, identified, or renewed intention) to step forward into the world, or not, as you and they are ready, willing, and able. Consider entering into confidential conversations with the Divine, the Mother Earth, and the Father Sky-Sun. Tell these beings about your little secrets and special creations…your precious mullings of spirit, and offer these sacred ornaments of your soul for sharing and blessing…to the rains, snows, winds, rock and fire people, the ones who crawl and wiggle, the winged-ones, the four-leggeds, the ones that swim, the one-celled ones, and the ones that have no name, *first*.

Hold your power and vision for a time, as long as possible. Allow it to nourish and replenish spent dreams and systems. There will be plenty of energy from the Divine current connection to publish and gift to the world, in a timely manner that will unfold and reveal its own emergent rhythm…itself an interesting thing.

SPIRIT TALK

So builds the myth, and the ever-renewed and recreated myths of partnered Creation and co-Creation. We are the new myth makers.

Bama mine,
Dawn Woman
Posted at 7:29 CST

Sunday, April 15, 2012

Gratitude Principle Teaching, Day 12

BozHo nikan,

Release…

SPIRIT TALK

Now is a good time to bring the fullness of *release* forward and continue on your/our ceremonial journey, at this time, of thinking all about life.

Bama mine,
Dawn Woman
Posted at 5:40 CST

Monday, April 16, 2012

Gratitude Principle Teaching, Day 13
Release...and Coming Forth

BozHo nikan,

Visit and consult the "grateful place." Consider proposing and inviting a joint "medicine journey" to certain "inner ones"...in the interest of furthering and guiding extended release activities, inviting and walking the twenty-one-day Gratitude Principle Ceremony into your/our larger world. The Natural World is a blessed place to visit and to sponsor special introductions of those gentle intentions, prayers, hopes, plans, wonderings, and knowings—the natural world that the Grandmother Moon calls home. Step out into the sunset and visit the western evening sky and make an offering-greeting to the Grandmother Moon, who is already wearing her new robes and showing her face to us.

Make a giveaway of greetings with your name, send love and acknowledgement of this "one" who lights our nights, governs the tides and the seasons...this "one of growing newness" who is walking with us at this time—the Spring and Planting Time. *Talk with her! Tell her your things!*

SPIRIT TALK

And so, in this Way as visionary farmers, tenders, and gardeners of our lives, we take this time to bring "our" special new ones forward to *Release, Join,* and *Unify* with the universal Giveaway and begin a renewed Dance of Life.

Let's go! It is good. It is very, very good.

Bama mine,
Dawn Woman
Posted at 5:48 CST

Tuesday, April 17, 2012

Gratitude Principle Teaching, Day 14
Star Walkers and Sweetgrass Burners

BozHo nikan,

From this day comes a special "remembering" point to bring forward. You have invested much into your interior Creation of self. There has been consent and surrender to investigation, purification, visioning, and construction of the "eternal present." The past, present, and future planes are concurrently occupying an interior space and reality shrouded in luminosity and radiance. Be breathed.

SPIRIT TALK

From this w/holy and sacred labor we remember love…Reseat in the "grateful place," drape yourself in the sacred color, speak your name and prepare to step forward, as we discover ourselves as the Divine Radiant Being we know ourselves to be.
    Enjoy all.

My love,
Dawn Woman
Posted at 5:35 CST

Wednesday, April 18, 2012

Gratitude Principle Teaching, Day 15

BozHo nikan,

The remaining seven days of the twenty-one day cycle are Spirit days. You may have, or will, forget the recent teachings and practices. I hope you have and will. This is the way it goes. You will remember on the twenty-first day, and the twenty-one-day Gratitude Principle Teaching will be complete. Cultivation of your Divine Inner Garden is in place and ongoing.

Understanding will be broadened and a peaceful atmosphere will pervade. You will be in a different place from where you began the twenty-one-day gratitude walk.

Bama mine,
Dawn Woman

Gratitude Principle Teachings, Day 16–20
Silent Spirit Days

The Spring Mother Earth's silent meditation awakening completes the Winter silent meditation—the time when the Mother Earth sleeps. Revisit Day 5 of Winter Quiet Time and allow it to nourish the seasonal awakening.

Gratitude Principle Teachings, Day 21
Completion

Bozho Nikan,

This day, rest, and at some point think about making a review of the previous outlines of the twenty-one-day Gratitude Principle Teachings. You might consider printing out the teachings... including any photos you took, personal reflections, art, pressed flowers, fabric swatches of your color, coffee rings, or grease spots,...or writings, and investing the teachings in a personal guidebook, which you may be inspired to expand with time. Slip the pages and photos into a plastic-spined presentation folder. Have some *fun* with it! *Laugh!*

SPIRIT TALK

This day concludes our interactive portion of the twenty-one-day ceremony. From this time forward, move intuitively forward in fine attunement with body, mind, heart, and Spirit, until we meet again to sit in spirit or actual circle and reflect for one another. The following seven days are yours to write. At some point within that time you may, or will, forget that you are within the twenty-one days…this is good. It has been internalized and is complete…only then you realize, with a start, that *it is now!* The twenty-first day.

Until then…*Migwech, wewene kiche migwech.*

Bama mine,
Dawn Woman
Posted at 5:29 CST

SPIRIT TALK

We have gathered our thoughts, hearts, and intentions; exchanged creative energies; seeded love and fellowship; and radiated, once again, to the four winds. The intention is completed…and the new cycle is initiated, with gratitude.

Kiche migwech, wewene kiche migwech,
Thank you, thank you very much (*Bodewadmin,* Potawatomi),
Dawn Woman

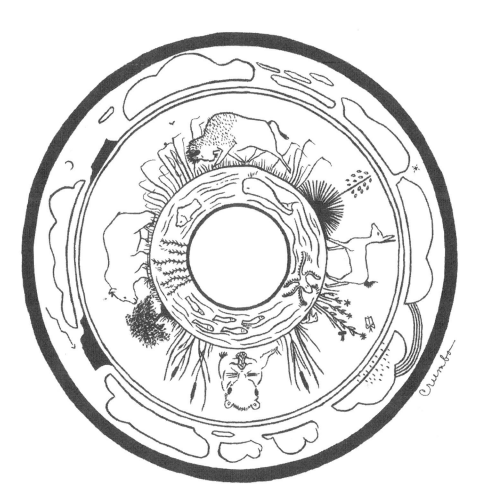

Circle of Life

The Circle of Life, as the water flows, the grass grows, and the winds blow:
there is beauty above, beauty below, beauty all around.
Deer stands at the East, direction of illumination and mental clarity—Spring.
Mouse stands at the South, direction of innocence and new life—Summer.
Bear stands at the West, direction of introspection and heart-felt gratitude—Fall.
Buffalo stands at the North, direction of wisdom and purity—Winter.

Circle of Life
Minisa Crumbo

SUMMER...NIBNEK

Revisit the White Plain,
Wisdom Ancestor and Pure Spirit Lover
of Innocence

Blackberry Winter, Mkedémen

By the white emergent flowers of earliest summer, genesis and kinship calls for a recollection of all previous significant begats. No season properly begins without first recalling the genealogy of those who came before, their contributions, attributes, and our relationships to the named ancestors.

Look around, call and write the names of all living things within eyesight. Make other lists. These are our relations.

THE FOUR CHIEF BERRIES

Démen—Strawberry
Mkedémen—Blackberry
Minen—Blueberry
Mskomen—Raspberry

By the emerging white in the summer morning sky, we are reminded of the winter white and the white flowers of the Blackberry Spring, which bloomed during the last cold snap in the middle back of Turtle Island, our home.

We think also of the white strawberry flower emerging from northern woodland snow blankets to bring forward the first sacred berry of the spring, strawberry, the démen. Good medicine.

BLACKBERRY WINTER

The white flowers of blackberry winter which often bloom around Easter presage another sacred berry, the blackberry, *mkedémen,* whose flowers appear as the final cold, hard male rains fall from the loosened bony fingers of that mean old man of the north. His grip is loosened and weakened at last by the warming airs, as he retreats with his sickness bundle just steps ahead of the soft, encouraging female rains. Finally, for some, the honey-tears, stiffened by cold, begin to soften and flow, sending streams of honeyed-held-back tears flowing…in shiny candy sheets.

The genesis, the calling of the names and the initiation of anything, but especially a new season, can be an unpredictable, mixed, and rocky time. We run forward, all full of anticipation. And then, we may be drawn up short by late and extreme weather events, transitions, mysterious pauses, voids, and vacuums, and thus slowed in the run for summer, we recall that perhaps, we must work for, remember, earn, and deserve to receive the full and knowing bounty of the sentient world. White dawn light comes slowly out of the night, accompanied at times by *guna gish pi,* the morning star sister of the east, which is to appear later in the year as the evening star.

DAWN @ THE RANCH

Dawn Woman, traveler of the morning twilight, the morning "crack between the worlds" that brings a twilight blue of limpid air, a mirror reflecting still water reflecting everything—macaw feathers and iridescent mallard heads, the blue-gray sea stones of Anatolian chalcedony, the pebble strewn beaches of Lake Michigan agate, and the wild slough flags. All these things and, more slowly, accept the first sweeping breezes of dawn and the sudden orange gilt of the rising sun.

SPIRIT TALK

Dawn Woman helps us to remember how to enter a room, to prepare for and receive a day, a season, and a life.

Summer Arrives

But first, we remember the white winter Spirit and the golden spring, the spiritual and mental antecedents, the energetic origins of dream and seed conceptions. Upon arriving at the edges of summer, the organization of the first template of Medicine Wheel polarity begins to reveal the first three of the four arms of its design. The white winter Spirit is a form, albeit very different in appearance and function from the mental and all other planes. The form of Spirit is so open and clear, so much more connected and more a part of the ethers that it can only be known and sensed, however, that does not make it any less active and effective, quite the contrary. Within the white winter Spirit is located a core source energetic transformer, a crystalline locus of intentional and random thought forms and histories. This locus receives, broadcasts, and transforms incoming and outgoing beingness particles, as they interface with the whole structure of the Medicine Wheel, an amplifying, dispersing, balancing, and purifying agent at the frontier of consciousness. It is formless form, but as such it is still a real place that can hold, stabilize, and support a being, activity, or concept in the flow of a current stream of activity—a positive transmuting accessory force of the white winter Spirit. The constancy, durability, and reliability of white winter Spirit and its source originator are our original partner, lover, and companion of our spirit. All of the time we spent at the altars of white winter purity and wisdom, as we fired the seeds of inspiration for this new year, has passed through the stern gauntlet of the golden spring fires and now, the white plain of winter marries the red mouse of summer innocence, bringing forward and delivering the winter dowry. Never, are winter and summer so close. Now, the Good Red Road that connects the north, purity and wisdom of winter, and the south, loving innocence of summer, begins to be forged for our Earth walk…an inner marriage of the Medicine Wheel. Balance meets and crosses with harmony and the Medicine Wheel engages in a summer marriage of essences, and the great gift itself is renewed.

Visit with these concepts, and consider making your own marriages with them when ready by entering into the locus, the Spirit center of the white winter wisdom or of the Medicine Wheel center. You may make the choice of another direction like the south to enter from, but at some point, consider visiting them both to see how they differ and how they meet in the center. Do this with the fullness of your being. Introduce yourself as the being of beauty, unity, and loving kindness that you know yourself to be. Take all of the uninterrupted time available to conceive and assemble an offering worthy of both yourself and the Creator Spirit, and bring it forward. Allow it to be received. Do not be surprised or dismayed if you find that the offering is actually you, yourself. This happens often, and what more worthy offering could ever be brought forward than our precious selves? When that has settled and calm is restored (with a high, thin layer of excitement) allow a perceived concern, issue, or challenge of the moment to mindfully enter with you, into the white-wisdom-purity locus with highest intention for all concerned, within a spirit of purity—a willingness of heart, flexibility, trust, courage, and endurance—that Creative resolution and transmutation can permeate, broadcast, or reintegrate the marriage energies through the spirit of crystalline balance and harmony.

Work this out for yourself. Trust. This is but one approach, the findings that follow, that you can own, live, and grow by. This is a place that can be called a home and a true Way…a Way by which we can conduct a tardy but well received self-initiation into Spirit knowingness. One need never again sit outside the door of Spirit, for this is but one of many Ways and paths by which man and womankind can close, or begin to close, the perceived sense separation with the Creator, and come to recognize and experience ourselves as a viable aspect of the Divine, to move into and live within the center of our unity consciousness, as we know it, and thereby, come to know the Mind of God.

In this Way, through the blood, sweat, tears, love, dream, and effort, we find our own Way, forging the personal good medicine by which we can live and die, feeling trust and confidence through the ways of breath, water, fire, wind—the Medicine Wheel, the Mother Earth and the Father Sky-Sun.

Upon arriving at this recognition, remembrance, and gratitude point, the summer joining-point in our journey upon and within the Medicine Wheel, the red mouse face of the southern Mother Earth's journey, we enter into a balance point with our opposite, the winter medicine, where we began so recently, to dream much of what we see now manifesting, which originated upon and within the white plain of winter wisdom and purity.

She Gives Away that New Life Might Come

Stepping within the threshold of each seasonal moment and entering our unique and personal portal rabbit holes of perception and experience, our medicine grows as we watch. The act of stepping within these thresholds implies presence of known medicines of proven and worthy value, as well as the unknown medicines. This will require the sharpening of all observing and knowing senses. These senses, when married to fine intention, proven and worthy values, are carried forward, and the new marriages call for many things, among them a change of raiment and sometimes a complete change, a giveaway metamorphosis of epic and courageous proportions like cocoon to pupa to...something else. A change of clothing...a time to change the coat...A time to adjust to the new normal..."Be breathed" and remember to express, if not feel, gratitude, until new understandings are reached and balance and harmony *begin* to be restored.

Taking Off the Coats

The medicine journeys may gradually or quickly reveal to us the coats of many colors we are called upon to accept, spin, weave, stitch, grow, barter for, or forge in order to move in alignment and fine attunement with the exigencies and requirements of each season and the events encountered there. But trust that revelations of these truths will and do arrive despite willingness or readiness to see or know.

Many are the truths displayed by distinctive garments, shields and armors, raiment; paints, tattoos, scarifications, and adornments that we, and others will wear as the seasons pass. Recalling our past relationships with the natural world will assist us in seeing, knowing, and correctly interpreting the weights and colors of ours or another's coat, paint, or skin. What is the message, the history, the need or desire that is now being made visible in the innocent red mouse face of the southern sun? Will it now be a shedding or molting? Now a giving off of pollen? Now a growth of thorn, a thickening foot pad? Taking a mate or giving birth? Spooling into elderhood? Grieving a loss? Seeking a cool and shady tunnel, drowning in flooded ground and rising water? Illness, lameness, loss of teeth? Rapid growth and maturity... shrunken, contracted, or attenuated opportunity...These seasonal and activity-drawn coats, valuable and necessary as they may have been and perhaps still are, will all eventually change and be outgrown as the marriages with each season are arranged and accepted. The old coats will be seen to peel away in their time, for what seed or bud did but arrive with a hard, tightly protective sheath, soon to split, open, and peel away, as moisture and heat does swell and cause to grow the prayed-over seed to emerge, that new life might come, smiled over and blessed by the Creator, our elemental parents, the natural world, and one of the prime systems on the planet, the Medicine Wheel Teachings.

For these and all things we are grateful. We are become as the loving innocence of the red/green mouse of the south, whose lover is the white breath of wisdom and purity, and at whose right and left sit the friendship of the golden east and the midnight blue of medicine introspection…and so many others. We are always becoming…

SPIRIT TALK

The mouse people sit in the medicine direction of the south. These summer people represent and teach the gentle qualities of innocence and love…their shadow face is fear. They move close to the Mother Earth upon their fine tiny feet and see the minutest details of their grassy homes and burrows and perceive the truths of the white plain, in this and all seasons, that all fear might be transformed and transmuted into love and trust.

Sweet, sweet summertime!

May 2 at 9:15 CST

Summer Represents Undeniable Progressive Evolution and Unity with All of Creation

The effects and evidences of ongoing life, whether intended or unintended, are evidenced everywhere. The invitations, solemnizations, and notices of marriage agreements and graduation ceremonies are flying through the air as summer-snows heavy with import. Heavy paper envelopes, bearing embossed script and seal, and weighty e-mail messages bid us take notice not only of what is accomplished but also, dually, that which is transitioning and passing away...Of histories streaming behind bearing the gathered warp and woof threads and spirit lines into tied-off and trimmed tassels, as carefully trimmed umbilicus marks and charges the newly departed child from its womb home of recent old, to "be breathed" on its own behalf by the Creative breath. Thus, we find ourselves suddenly deposited into and occupying the long sought after, and striven for, days and nights of the red-greenness of the earthen southern summer. Being dropped rather suddenly and precipitously into the new, we hasten to give shape to this "new," which has been so zealously sought. We hasten also to search for new meanings, refocus, to fix aim on horizons and destinations so long seen in the distance and then, upon arrival, to appear as rawly foreign arrivistes demanding an attention we may suddenly find ourselves unprepared to receive.

It is suddenly time to slow down and catch up with that which has been wrought, fashioned, dreamed, prayed over, carried over, and inherited from our recent, busy, and oh, so carefully tended fields of white winter and golden spring yearnings now becoming cloaked in the new raiment of summer.

The longer suns and spring rains of May Day, may find us dancing into fecund fields of manifested potential and cheerful evidences of positive evolution, but even the day knows the night for rest and restoration. The warm night soil temperature propagates and encourages the strong rootlet and stem establishment of tender plants and animals still lashed by the stern wake-up calls of the walking male rains. Each bright sunrise is a renewed altar call to life, each sunset, a return to the dark embrace of the warmed lover, the altar of deep inner remembrance...night, a time when all things are protected...Young turkeys and geese, young children of the two-leggeds, young sweet peas carrying young in their own new blossom, young tender green leaves and grasses, tadpoles, freshening springs and streams; calves, impossibly wide-mouthed young birds in the nest, and all young hopes and dreams…all come forward bravely and exuberantly bearing unfurling banners of personal history and dynamic intent, spreading green pollen dust clouds and manifold bird "calls to action." Sleep we must, pace and speed we must, remember we must.

Birth

Visionary Separations and Creations

The renewal of succeeding seasons and our "walks" with them, as well as our works and rededicated efforts to host the continuance of new life forms, can and perhaps will bring a certain need to pause and reflect. Energetic efforts to correctly assess the space and time needs while mindfully creating and then dedicating real ceremonial and ritual continuum is necessary, in order to maintain pace with the sometimes slow, sometimes rampant growth the early summer experiences. Consider it also a very real possibility that the rapid departures and growth spurts may and will create a certain potential vacuum that will pose as deep fatigue, but may in reality mask a "post-partum" depression or let down. As with any being that bears reproductive life, when that new life reaches its evolutionary goals, recognizing and occupying them, angst and separation anxieties then exist alongside feelings of satisfaction and the celebration of successful vision and conception completions. Birth is a mixed and complex transitional time. We experience these diverse and dual activities as surely as the plant, weather, animal, and spirit beings do. We meet them in field, water, and air for they are the meat and potatoes of duality, the principle system by which the Creator Spirit and ourselves have chosen to manifest as Spirit Beings within physical bodies at this time.

The Duality System

The duality system is powerfully and forcefully demonstrated on ours and all other life forms at all times but is *very* compellingly so in the "manifestation of dream" time, within the red or green colors of the southern summer. The prayerful and serious attention that was brought to bear upon and within our lives during the "firing the seeds of inspiration" time, white northern winter, and the "new life comes" time of the golden eastern spring are the *conception* and *initiating* blocks of the Medicine Wheel. The third and fourth blocks are *abundance* and *harvest*, thus completing the circle.

The "separation anxieties" we perceive as new season cycles evolve, as well as the "celebrated and joyful blossomings," are one of the earmarks, or identifications, of the duality system... opposites and pairs conceived and perceived coming together to make a marriage producing new life. That's the Way it is with us now. This is the central message by which we all live at this time, within the eye and mind of Prime Creator. We have but to accept, surrender, survive, embrace, honor, and...finally, celebrate this fine and distinct system of creative manifestation. However finely and divinely conceived this system we shall call duality, the Divine Labors are manifestly apparent and yes, demanded, of each and every one of us in the here and now.

Each and every being-one of us must find and eternally *renew* the vision and strength to conceive, remember, and hold the myriad visions of new life, to give or allow new life to emerge bearing a large measure of our own life force as "start-up" fuel and to survive the emergent division. This emergent division *is* the physical, energetic mimic of the principal perception of separation anxiety that is present in most, if not all, spirit entities, as they emerge from the spirit pool of the Creator. The perception of separation pain is then the origin of all other projected fear, sorrow, and pain and must be "doctored" by appropriate action.

Summer Ceremonies

The Doctorings

And since many, or most, of us do not live in close proximity to adepts and holy people that can and do facilitate community ceremonies, that appropriate action is, in the end, essentially personal. So what matters is bringing the fullness of our minds, hearts, bodies, and spirits forward to say *yes* once more to life. Herein and from this point on, we are offered the opportunity for which we were born, that of recognizing ourselves as our *own* holy people. *Aho!*

Take up the staff of authority and don the mantle of leadership, and if you will, emerge and embark upon finding, forging, and designing a Way that is unique to your personal attributes and needs. These are the new Ways coming forward for the new days...and we are the ones. Since each of us initially think principally upon ourselves, as it should be, let us now think even more and deeply upon ourselves and the personal links to what we can identify as the proven and worthy gifts of life, the Sacred and all of its auspices. This is a deeply personal and sacred moment to be held close, in silence and privately, for some time to mature and seat in the deepest, innermost recesses of your sacredness. Take time for the building of this precious personal medicine, our personal medicine treasure—that of which we know and that of which we are—together and in a spirit of oneness with the mind of the Creator, in concert with these first, most beautiful and enduring gifts to and for us from the Creator: our Mother the Earth, our Father the Sky-Sun, our Grandmother the Moon, our relations: the Star People, the Directions, the Elementals, the Spirit Helpers, the colors, the Wind Beings, the Fire Beings, the Green Beings, the Water Beings, the Stone People, and all of the other named and unnamed sacred related beings that live upon and within this beautiful Creation.

The old people say, "That which you recognize, you own."

They also say, "It's not so much, will you *do* it, but whether you will *remember* to do it."

First Steps

Divine and design some physical time from which to create and dedicate a personal internal meeting place where the continuums of the previous winter and spring can be brought forward, honored once again, and remembered with gratitude. And only then, can it truly be integrated into the *now* of Summer, making a complete, healed and whole fabric, woven of the highest potential and the hardest of realities: the births and the deaths, screaming happiness and silent disappointment, rank feelings of separation and sweet, bee pollinated flower thrusts to make, honored seed beings and scant resources, the whole gamut of transitions…All possibilities present and accounted for…bring it *all* in and allow it to be.

Now, y'all come on into the circle and be counted. The great summer ceremonies are *all* healings and honorings like this, some way or another, and the only one that can and will speak truly to and of each one of us, is of our own heart and design whereby we can *begin* to close and to dispel the perception of separation between ourselves and the Creator…And, to put an *end* to all that is not *real*.

This day, or soon, create a space within which to sit, think, and design a personal ceremony. Draw a Circle of Life on the ground, or floor, and *move within it*…Metaphorically or physically, alone or with others, begin to dance, drum, sing, burn incenses and fragrant dry herbs, take a ritual bath of cornmeal, smile, listen to music, sweat, work, talk, heal, look, rest, pet the pet, pass the talking stick, feast later and feed the precious mind, heart, body, and spirit with all good and desirable things. No shame, no blame...take some time to mark these passages of the hours and days in which we pass through the divinely constructed and offered Gift of Life within this consciously designed Circle of Gratitude.

And now, we are progressing into the sweet summer of the direction of the south, the restored and renewed path of innocence and love.

And so, the voids and vacuums become filled, emptied, cleaned, and purified through the choice, imperative, due dates, and gifts of the seasons as they appear.

May 2 at 9:44 CST

With remembrances, honorings, and conceptions. In this and in many other Ways does life go on "in a good way."

Dawn Woman Comes

Dawn Woman, Wabaksekwe, comes on the edge of the morning twilight, the blue-white light of the new day. She comes on the twilight of the late dream. She comes quietly and easily to light the initiate's new day.

This past twenty-one days as we made our ingress into the innocence and love and the direction of the southern summer, by the natural calendar, have been a mixed number of days, bringing forward that which has been prayed over from the winter and spring, that within which we live and the anticipated bounty of the sweet, sweet summertime.

If you will recall, the natural world marks the yearly cycle every three months, starting with the spring day/week of January 21st (notably referred to as the spring thaw). The succeeding seasonal cycles are concluded and initiated every three months on the third week, on or around the 21st of the month.

The previous chapter is a spring count of days, marking and charting some of the energetic possibilities of that season. It could as well have been a winter or autumn count of days. Often, the first twenty-one days of ingress into a new season may be viewed as the dawn of the season. As with the late dark and early twilight, all may not yet be clear. The lines of the hand may not yet be visible but are known. This is a good time to meditate and set the path of the day by making and offering supportive prayers to our Mother Earth, as she pushes to give birth to yet another day.

May 4 at 24:04 CST

New Life Comes

We have made all of the preparations we can think of, observances, propitiatory and celebratory ceremonies, purchases, giveaways, and date-book entries possible. The first steps, looks, and intuits into the new season are complete, used up and over. It is now time load up the gains, gifts, and visions, to step out of the heavily self-referenced initiatory stages and merge these gifts and gains with the larger world.

Like a hot iron skillet, well-oiled and heaped with thinly sliced onions, the sizzle begins. All of the diverse elements from the shop, pantry, water well, desk, field, mine, Facebook inspiration, campfire, or windmill will surge and measure from our hands, creating new normals, stabilizing and exhilarating, within the skillet as they flow inbounds and outbounds...new life comes.

Good Medicines of the Body

Like the first wild greens, roots, and fruits—raw, strong and sweet—the earliest emerging plants and foods are designed to purify, strengthen, and thin the blood in preparation for summer's heat. The wild onion is cooked or steamed with eggs or ground meat, the thrice-boiled poke salat greens (the first and second waters are uncongenial and must be poured away), the sassafras root tea (parent of the root beer beverage), the tiny wildwood strawberry drink brings "good medicine" for women and men, white dandelion greens, saguaro cactus flowers, maple sap running, eggs, horseradish and salt offerings, mushrooms… are all harbingers and early substantial proofs that life will and does go on.

These medicines live on in us for, like breath, we cannot "take" life. We receive life and are lived in concert with all of Creation. What are the Mother Earth medicines where you live? Make another list.

Good Medicines of the Mind and Spirit

These medicines are more than foods, these medicines are gifted to shift and alter our perspective and experience. They enter into the dedicated spaces we create, bringing strengthening and purifying physical energies, solar intelligence, new formats and codes designed to update and stock the existing wisdom and knowledge we have inherited, built, observed, been taught, and accrued. This information is then received and relayed to the appropriate inner shelving for immediate or future processing and retrieval. Proper shelving is essential or much incoming information will continue moving quickly into and on out of passing consciousness. Much information will be noted and understood, but here we come to that saying of the old people, "It's not so much will you *do* it as, will you *remember* to do it?"

Let us use the word "shelving" for simplicities sake, although the words filing, stocking, or storage may come to mind for this activity. Select a word of choice by which you personally identify the concept of retention and retrieval of items deemed worthy of keeping, further study, contemplation or mediation, active experimentation, examination or use, and at least temporarily worthy of more than passing consideration.

Building, Shelving, and Initiating it

The concept of shelving is important and essential. Shelving is part and parcel of thorough support and retention in early childhood development and training. Societies and cultures worldwide that have accepted and forged an external workplace model (school) or an internal model of initiation practices have fine-tuned education for very specific purposes.

However, tribal and indigenous societies strive to retain values selected from principal identification and introduction with the natural world and relationship with the Creator and living world of spirit and flesh through cultural frameworks, such as the Medicine Wheel Teachings and other constructs. The shelving to receive and retain this information and experience is laid down early in life, and then specifically through training or initiation rites on or around puberty. This practice is a continuance of guided and supported ways that are relevant to the family or culture of origin and serve to create and maintain vital connection to the identified Creative Source of birth, or later, choice. This then, is the juncture where many of us now find ourselves. Relevance is the issue.

The juncture of the self-initiation of choice by the mature adult, hence the deep inner explorations of what we would find most desirable, necessary, and meaningful for establishing a personally sound, morally ethical, balanced, sensitive, loving, and successful platform upon which to observe, live, grow, evolve, and to ultimately make a fearless and unified physical transition into Spirit.

Should you elect to seek your personal relevancies and findings regarding the unpaved paths and unwritten pages of the later-in-life initiation, read on. Recognizing ourselves and others as our own holy people in the sacred act of seeking, divining, finding, forging, and living a Blessing Way, is recognized and seen to be good. And now, to begin the radiantly compelling, attentive and spirit-filled path of the new mystic! Always, the now...for that is what we have—the eternal present.

Breathing and Being

Make your most serious and heartfelt prayers and offerings around these thoughts, bathe in and offer the sacred herb smoke...and take your time, all you need. Some people like to think and dream in four-day increments, some seven, some twenty-one, or twenty-four hours. Visit and interact normally with others while waiting, watching, and listening. Write, sing, fast, read, go to work, paint, cook, break down and rebuild a tranny, feast, exfoliate and pare the nails, dance, chant, sweat, sleep, examine the dreams, throw the I Ching, consult a black beetle, look at wasp nests, read your astrology, draw a Medicine Wheel on the earth with a stick, enter within it, facing the direction that feels best and ask, "What do I really want?" In the end, let all findings take their places and look to see what remains in your heart of a proven and worthy nature, what remains and lives in your heart for you and the highest good of all concerned...all of Creation. Have you had a good time and allowed yourself to simply *be?*

Ahora!...Enter the Now and invite the now to enter the heart center, to rest and in time, come to radiate and irrigate the entire being of mind, heart, body, and spirit, naturally, quietly, calmly, and even unnoticed. You may, if you choose to, consider and recognize this to be the first move of the new initiate, who now has some fresh new shelving to install and items to be entered on the shelves. (*Be Here Now.* Thanks, Ram Dass!)

This shelving, or another design which you may conceive, may be viewed as occupying the center, spokes, and circle(s) of your personal Medicine Wheel. Observe where this center sets up. It may be in the heart center, the mind, the solar plexus, or another location, preferably within your physical body. If you do find that it appears to be outside of the physical body, gently and lovingly invite it to shift, or begin shifting, residence to the heart center. This may take some time but it is important that this move takes place as soon as possible. Now, having located this center, honor it with smiling gifts of welcome, recognition, and gratitude. This center and all related positions within and adjacent to your Medicine Wheel will, from this point in time, be known and be the true home of the ever fresh, vibrant, and spirit-filled cosmos of yourself, the newly recognized self-initiate, mystic. Yes, you can rejoice for you have accomplished/are accomplishing this for yourself in partnership with the Creator Spirit and your natural parents and relations. Future gifts of value and items of interest now have a dedicated structure upon which to seat and to be available for full, accurate, and immediate retrieval.

The absence or incomplete nature of appropriate initiatory and/or guidance activities toward forming essential ways by which to think, creatively track the mind, and to function in friendly connection with necessary information and the collective knowledge of how to implement this knowledge reveals itself in many negative and painful social histories. Who among us has not cried for a word of wisdom and a crumb of understanding and knowledge,…for we know ourselves be capable of so much more. These and other ways are some time-tested Ways by which we can come, or begin to come, into fine attunement with ourselves, the larger world, and the Prime Creator, the Master of All Breath. Let us never forget that we are the Sacred.

The structures suggested in this text and others you know of, or will discover, are built upon and superimposed upon the firmest of foundations, the great Medicine Wheel of the Mother Earth and the Father Sky-Sun. So it has been from the first days of your birth and so it is now, the *birthright* of all sentient and non-sentient beings.

The prayed over and fired seeds of winter's inspiration... continue their journey. The refreshed, inspired, and illuminated seeds of all inherited previous harvests are sprouting.

We are the farmers of our lives and *now!* New life comes. *Aho!*

New Life Comes,
Maintaining and Functioning,
from the Sacred Center of Balance and Harmony,
the Arms and Trunk of the Medicine Wheel.

May 4 at 17:42 CST
Re: Summer and Autumn Notes

Knowing Beauty

Life is mostly about maintenance. Much of the hard work is in the past. Once the conscious return to the spiritual home-center within is sought and accomplished, the sacred charge is the basically delightful work of holding as much attention as possible in this experience of balance, harmony, and beauty. It will require a new discipline. Many times in the past we have allowed thoughts and feelings to roam free rein, often making returns to negative associations, histories, attractions, habitual attitudes, or passive negative associations that are hoped to further feelings of solidarity with an individual or group mind-set. Hosting negativity will hinder—guaranteed—the building and maintenance of the fullest life experience of a new mystic.

Watch the thoughts like an eagle. Upon identifying undesirable, unloving, depressive, angry, fearful, controlling, or manipulative, jealous, vengeful, or sorrowful thoughts, acknowledge and honor them. Pull the weeds of the Divine Garden. Maintenance. Aspire also to learn the content and meaning of their message and immediately, or as soon as possible, direct and return them to the great reservoir of spirit energy, where they will be purified and renewed. Release them to make their own blessing journey and return to Source, sending them on their return path with gratitude and love, on the breath as well as thought. The eyes can also direct releases, with permission, to the clouds. The breath, being the constant link with life and the Divine is ever present, able, and willing to transmute and transform into Spirit, that which is truly dead, dying or diseased...no longer wanted or needed. Be sure that only ones personal business is addressed. At all times be observant of others' sacred and psychic privacy and freedom of choice. Maintaining a respectful mien, which is increasingly built by *mindful*, positive choices and growing awarenesses of *what* and *how* we think, act, and intend *at all times,* is essential. This practice of thorough attention is a cumulative, life process and will grow more robust with practice and the seasons, so move forward and regularly provide the sweet water of loving kindness to the young Sacred Flowering Tree, and to the young *skebyak*, the green beings, born of the same elemental parents as ourselves. What kind of tree or shrub are you?

Now, how does it go again? Would you remember...To return and re-center within the center of the Sweet Medicine home of balance, harmony, and beauty whenever necessary and to resume functioning from this place? As time goes by, and many of these suggestions are being considered and possibly entertained, some of you may envision alternate places and ways, other words or systems, customs, and traditions. At the same time, these highest aspirations may also open heretofore only previously dreamed of and hoped for thresholds to planes and levels of expanded growth, radiant and unified experience, inspired and illuminated truths…to the new mystic.

May 5 at 11:28 CST

Walking the Good Red Road

The path is now well laid, open and ready to be traversed. Grounded and drenched as we are in the full grip of the summer sap rain, we feel the invitation to walk, look, listen to the beckoning Good Red Road that connects the north-south energies of purity and wisdom with those of innocence and love. It is timely now to broaden these anchoring qualities and directions, releasing the intensely subjective work of late. Soften and release the highly focused, organized and disciplined study of the mental Medicine Wheel, direction of the east, and open the floodgates of the emotional heart center. Carry forward the dazzling solar lover of the mind and the pristine pure spirit lover of wisdom, and issue to them an irresistible invitation to step forward into a foot stomping, dipping and swooping, shoutin', callin', an' whistle-blowin' circle dance. There now, we are happening. The marriage talks are gaining momentum, consummation is in the wings, radiance, fulfillment, and love "are dancing outside our window." (Thanks, Buffy Sainte-Marie.) Sweet fruits are forming out of joy and abandon.

The cool and distilled winter breath issues a full exhalation remembrance of original purity and wisdom to hasten the seeds so recently fired with inspiration…the inspiration is now stepping its own inspired dance around the Medicine Wheel. Purity joined with love, *aahhh*, the beauty. Wisdom hand in hand with innocence rocks the mind and rolls the body.

And, this then, is an aspect of the Good Red Road: love and innocence, connecting with the purity and wisdom, braided into the Earth walk. A treasure both ethereal and incorporate—a divine light, core home center, turning eternally within the full known and unknown brilliance and possibility of the finite and infinite great Medicine Wheel of life.

Endeavor to create a space in time to visit and seat the Good Red Road and make a dance! Live in the light.

Scanning the Horizon

When autumn, the time of the physical and introspection arrives, a full stop, four-way crossroad will emerge. This road is called the hard road of life, because it originates out of and connects the eastern mental plane with that of the western physical plane. All of these planes are necessary and desirable elements for creating and holding a paradigm of the duality experience. We shall visit this path, the hard west road of life, and explore it in due time as we complete this circumambulation and great crossroad of the Medicine Wheel cycle. None of these paths can really be avoided or lingered upon for long. Each path brings an aspect of growth and development appropriate to the direction. The time spent in each direction varies widely and may include concurrent directions, but principal visits to each direction may be expected to last approximately two-and-a-half years. The individual birth season will determine the basic affinity direction, however, the time of the first acquaintance reading of the Medicine Wheel will indicate where the individual now resides. Subsequent movements upon the Medicine Wheel are often in a continuous, clockwise (sun path) way, but not always. This will be for the walker to observe and discover...all of the clues and markers are to be found within the natural world, the seasons and the opportunities, necessities, and desires that come your way. Some of the perceived difficult or undesirable walks may not be avoided for long, or at all, and it is good to remember that often the only way out is all the way through. Read back, remember, pray for understanding and endurance, renew and purify, make smoke and food offerings and gifts...endeavoring always to *make* gratitude responses for everything until it becomes an automatic response. Return often to the eternal Center and allow present moment awareness to seat in gratitude and flow freely through your feelings, spirit and thoughts, until the *returns* last longer and longer and, finally, for always.

SPIRIT TALK

The radiant light center home of the Sacred Flowering Tree is where the paths cross, bringing all possibility to our door. It is all of these paths we must traverse, earning the competence and right to reside fully in the center of the Medicine Wheel, which then allows us to incorporate many of the directional qualities spoken and considered with these words. Unspoken of, because there are yet directions and mysteries unspoken to remain known only in Spirit Talk.

On May 4, 2014, at 20:41 CST

- Cultivating the Earthly Garden of the Direction of the South
- Planting, watering, fertilizing, weeding, and gathering
- Looking Toward and Entering Autumn—the Direction of Black Western Introspection
- The Hot-Dry-Wind walks with the Early Harvests
- July 21
- The first twenty-one days

Autumn: The Primary, Secondary, and Tertiary Division takes Final Shape and Form.

Autumn: The Fourth Quarter completes the Circle and makes a Whole.

May 7 at 13:09 CST

First there was Spirit.

Then Spirit organized into conceptual, linear and physical duality.

Duality found a home and expression upon and within another system, ours.

The Medicine Wheel is an independent but evolutionarily related, secondary, four-quarter, cellular division of linear duality, possessing a center and concentric circle-ringed divisions…

An eighth fold division exists. It is present in Spirit, silent, unseen and unspoken.

Cellular division continues until it must fold back into the linear, initiating the differentiation of species and subsequent specific development.

These interwoven lines, circles, and dots are the stuff and substance of creative material, crackling and moving in the fires, waters, airs, and ethers with variable lights, sounds, and electricity. They are the present and available primal building blocks of intention, generating wormholes of vibrant and positive awareness and consciousness track, demonstrating seen, and now unseen, evolutionary patterns and possibilities, without cease.

Early Autumn

The first twenty-one days of autumn can bear the mark of instability, as have the initial (initiation) twenty-one days of each previous season. Harvests of medicine and introspection bring happiness, a sense of accomplishment, and deep reflection upon that which has been wrought in the previous three seasons, recognitions of that which is certainly coming forward and revealing the fullness of itself. The past no longer is and the new is not yet.

Early autumn, a time to pause, reflect, to *be* in rest…before the foot turns to acquaintance with the west-east hard road of life.

Summer: This year's story is rapidly moving toward the Autumn-Harvest Story, but for now, the seed is still being made.

May 11 at 9:59 PM

Exploring the Essential Wildness of Life

After all the counting, selecting, planning, making, and firing of prayers, waiting, listening, cultivating of the Divine Inner Garden, preparing the physical beds, raking in aged sheep poop, drawing the rows and forming mounds, selecting and soaking seeds, waiting for and watching the Grandmother Moon's progress, last frosts, and finally with the putting in of new plants and the dropping in of wordless hopes and silently prayed over seeds, I am brought to release all of the effort and surrender to the essential wildness of life—my life and the whole carefully tended concept of thinking I knew even a little bit of what I was doing and what was happening!

The blast of summer medicine has rocked my world open to the vast and unknown potential that secretly, or not so secretly, I hope, dream, and pray will one day be restored, the liberty of the wild creative love and innocence.

So, if the messages of nature are not listened to, what will be listened to? The new will enter with all of the whole correctness set to unfold, unfurl, reveal, and return, moment to moment, to satisfy the original instructions, and any other use of energy will risk becoming a grave distraction and expenditure of energy.

Attention and energy, knowing the not known-ness of the evolved original face is the only worthy toil of the farmer's Divine Inner Garden, now finding itself in form.

Grasshoppers, the bane of my farmer's life have not appeared this year. I hesitate even to speak of it, but if they are part of the new myth,...the stories of plagues, droughts, floods and other unavoidable disappointments must be told. Their absence has opened up and relaxed all kinds of other stories—riotous stories. Laughter and song live in the rows this year. Life and love have returned to the rows. I know goodness this year.

The Salad Days...

Are upon us again. Tender lettuce leaves, asparagus spears, and early herbs, thrice washed, are already on the table. The cantaloupe, cucumber, and blue corn seeds are sprouting. The heirloom tomatoes are putting on their first blooms, the bok choy, hot chiles and sweet peppers, squash, and spring onions are stabilizing and strengthening. Wild things are happening in the garden...each plant having its own look and way. The returning arugula survivors are bolting early and preparing to phase out... others are poised to take over. And I do mean take over! I am ever and increasingly aware that the natural world is poised to over grow every inch of earth on this old, eroded Cretaceous hill here in the Cross Timbers country of Oklahoma upon which my husband, two dogs, and myself visit and live...as long as we might.

SPIRIT TALK

The night. The wind. I'm going to stay strictly centered for the moment and drift with the atmosphere, attentive to the power that is released when I listen and obey.

More later on the "take over" initiatives.

May 11 at 22:40 CST

The "Take Overs"

If we don't "go over" to the teachings of the natural world we're missing a prime evolutionary moment, for the human species is no longer in the ascendancy. Our projected paths have both narrowed precipitously and broadened radiantly. The choice is ours…actually there probably *is* no choice about whether we will successfully evolve in harmonious concert with the Mother Earth, only about the individual degree of personal choice one forms and occupies regarding participation.

Summer, it's gonna rain soon…

Today at 14:11 CST

The Good Red Road Establishes

Core dream and vision is about fullness of being, projects, and goals that will follow the seed into the prepared fertile furrows. Some seed beings will pass, some will fail, some will endure, and some will proliferate strongly and command more space, attention, and resources…taking over.

High summer on the Good Red Road is pregnant and giving abundant birth to the dreams and visions set forth by each of us as we sit by our fires, leafing through the seed catalogues of choice and intentionally, or unintentionally, setting much of what we see now, in place.

High summer recalls the winter marriage talk and agreements and now, the Good Red Road connecting the home direction of south: Heart, innocence, and love is built, in place and visible from where we originally sat or stood, and in the home direction of north: spirit, wisdom, purity, and breath. It is ours to walk. We built it according to original directions, persevered, and now we can stand back and look. The entire structure of the Medicine Wheel is almost completely assembled, but a toe-hold on even one small portion can give access to a rabbit hole threshold to another dimension of understanding, a dimension the powerful in spirit live in and draw from.

This would be a good time to revisit the Winter and Spring chapters. At this point in the initial movement (if it is your first movement) on the Medicine Wheel, so much has been assembled, initiated, experienced, and constructed that you may have forgotten more than you know. Living in the now can have that effect; hence the encouraging words "to remember." But then, as in many great progresses, the time comes when we must "apparently forget" everything and move forward, trusting that nothing of lasting value is lost and that the most proven and worthy of tools will accompany us forward. The esoteric "leaps of faith," forging the silent, invisible, and mysterious links between the known and the unknown, are taken as the rabbit hole threshold is crossed and information is accessed, renewed, or added, examined at leisure and stored in the Medicine pouch for the Winter Story Telling Time.

Spirit Talk and Responsible Spirit Duties

The medicine links and paths begin to take inner shape as individual, personal medicine grows in balance and harmony with the elemental parents, ourselves, and all of Creation. The big letters have become our norms. No more caps are necessary. The honorings are inherent and understood. The spirit talks are being spoken, felt, and heard…they can be observed, spoken of, questioned deeply, and stringently tested for efficacy and relevance. This is both a personal right and a duty. Take no word unquestioningly, be it the word of some unidentified "Spirit" entity, the random thought emanating from another person and drifting upon the ethers, any and all teachers, books, TV shows, flashes of smile or temper, any item of our own idle, unconscious or unpurified history, any disconnected or undisciplined function of our desire body, outright control or manipulation challenges that desire undue influence over ourselves or another, judgment responses without measure or investigation. Testing and proofing are called for on all fronts. If something cannot, or will not, tolerate or withstand deep scrutiny or question, take notice, be courteous, offer thanks, and immediately examine all available material and petition Spirit for additional, balanced, and true understandings by asking, "Spirit, what's going on here?"

Journal, chart, or record a daily progress, for within these evolutionary years we are in the act of writing the new calendars, myths, and histories. Date the entries. Identify them by other means, work and love interests of all kinds, art, weather, season and crop notations, singing, listening to or writing a song, animal movements, temperatures, colors, birthdays, anniversaries, promotions, stories, graduations, moves, clearing, adding, accumulating and releasing, transitions of all stripes. Looking back and revisiting this account of initiating these new years, times, teachings, and disciplines will reveal important patterns, cycles, and relevancies. The practice of personally noting and understanding cyclical ebbs and flows will not only reveal, they will help you be in a position to reinforce, build, and contribute and fuse coherent and desirable layers of fresh, new, and inspired personal vision to the proven and worthy tools of the natural world and the Medicine Wheel. By these ways do we increasingly come to recognize and to hear our true spoken gifts of the Creator and those of others,...and that is *us*, as well. We are *that*. For would we remember that which we are told, that we are created in the image of God?

It Rains, with Thunder, Wind, and Lightning

Now, the foot is set firmly upon the Good Red Road. Place both feet on it. Walk. The year's labor is bearing first visible fruit. Receive the fruits and enjoy them as a bee in flower, a wasp in fruit, a trout on frog egg, a bird on a worm…

The nectars of life are flowing through all of the tributaries of the wheel and most are sweet. There is yet, the gathering of much more abundance, so prepare and so make ready the additional shelving upon which to receive, catalogue, store, and retrieve, upon ready demand or need, the bounty and reserves which are registered at this time. Acknowledgement, appreciation, and enthusiasm are the coins of the realm, the fat, the gold of superfluous abundance, the milk and flowing honey, dripping down the chins of all living things. We will look back on this time when next we sit in another direction. Perhaps in the north where we can be found stoking the coming winter fires of wisdom and purity, sitting on the Good Red Road in the north, looking south. But, that is in the future. Core dream and vision continues to make its evolved movements from the summer marriages inexorably toward the direction of the west and season of the autumn harvest and leaves turning yellow. The *gishget*.

The Hard Road of Life Emerges as We Approach the West
The Roads Cross
The Sacred Flowering Tree Grows

But first, let us make and store the physical, spiritual, and metaphorical fats and begin to prepare for emergence into that still distant direction of the west, the black, physical, water, medicine direction of introspection where the Hard Road of Life is found that connects with the direction of the mental, fire, solar east. Like Eisenhower, we are building a new road system. Where those roads cross is where lives the Sacred Flowering Tree…We are that tree.

SPIRIT TALK

Core dream and vision arrive at and complete the Medicine Wheel Circle in the winter north to rest, restore, and begin anew, sitting in the north of the Good Red Road, looking south and remembering in song, story, dance, and dream.

The Thunder Beings speak. Aho! That is all.

May 14, 2014

The blueberry *minen* Full Moon

The *minen* ripen.

Full Moon feast suggestion: Gather berries "in a good way" and make a blueberry pie.

Dawn @ the Ranch

The Summer Rains

The rain falls on blue corn sprouts and marble-size tomatoes. It falls on last year's and the year before last's bolted arugula and already toughened mint. It falls on volunteer garlic, wild greens, and mullein started from last year's bloom. The Mullein Being I dug from the base of a pine tree outside of Flagstaff, Arizona, and carried back in a Styrofoam cup. The majestic Fibonacci spiraled cones and broad fuzzy medicine leaves thrive in the rich compost and watered kitchen garden, casting more seed and plant than I had bargained for on that fragrant day with the summer wind soughing through the pine canopy, and now I must deal with the abundance.

It is the medicine plant for soothing and healing sprained and broken bodies...limbs, skin, broken minds, and smoke-erupted lungs. More medicine than I can give away, tell of, store or transplant, so it must be a garden of healing the distant and unknown maladies.

Now, the sun has come out and the straight-down rain is falling harder. It will stop soon but there is more to come. We need you, western water beings, to run and gurgle down the afternoon pipes. The hollyhock growing from seed, gathered beside the Ranchos de Taos church with the painting of the Virgin Mary that begins to glow long after the lights are shut off, needs your water.

The mullein plants, recovering from the shock of transplant, need real water from the sky.

It stops now, the fast veil of rain that draws a medicine curtain between what was recently then…and now. Blessing and encouraging now, and the new.

With your permission, rain beings, we receive your gift of life and grow.

The rains are over for now and birds begin to sing again.

With the Mullein Beings, summer 2014

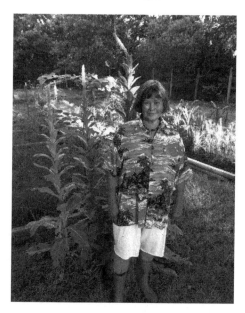

May 27, 2014, 14:16 EST

Building Trust, We Are Our Own Ancestors

A Memorial Day Tale:

Along with the acknowledged and manifold gifts and beauties of our world, we concurrently reside alongside many old, hard, and even ancient entities and energies that house upon, within and without, our beautiful Mother Earth. It is not to be taken for granted that they are intrinsically negative or dangerous, but as with anything powerful and unknown their territories and pathways must be negotiated with caution, respect, and as much conscious awareness as possible. The electric fan is unknown to the child and is essentially a benign tool of convenience until the child blindly and innocently sticks a finger into the moving blades. So, let us leave behind for now the unknown, the not necessarily bad but possibly negative to us, encounters with unknown or uncomfortable pathways and live in the present that we might be best prepared to deal with deeper issues with new and vibrant tools of understanding and acceptance as they arise.

Creator,
Prayers and Blessings of Gratitude Be With Us in This Teaching

Our world as we know it, and do not know it, is made up of multitudes of differing vibrations and frequencies and wavelengths. The intersections of these frequencies with our own is the material of miraculous encounters, prophesy, thought, vision, and dreams—the eureka moments. We willingly utilize and participate in and with these alternate and parallel levels, or layers, of differing realities unquestioningly when engaging in prayer, hopes, wishes, and goal making, indeed, planning of any kind. And we rely on the semi-mystical and fondly held dream potentials, and solidly inspirational clashes with which we view and endow them, to gain us entry, entertain our requests and, hopefully, grant us ingress or fulfillment of our goal and satisfaction.

The Medicine Wheel is a complete structure capable of containing all of the disparate elements of mind, heart, body, and spirit as we are given to know, trust, and understand them in the present moment. The core energetics of the Medicine Wheel Teachings are among the ancient, trusted, and creative tools that are one of the transferred patterns of the Creative Mind of Prime Creator and can be also be a creative tool of our own Earth walk. Our dreams, hopes, prayers, visions, initiatory activities, goals, and aspirations are groupings that can be made more visible, known, and maximized within this sacred space of our own and the relatively perceived mind of the Creator.

Occasions like anniversaries, weddings, birthdays, births, burials, household moves and job changes, planting and harvest observances, graduations, national holidays, and memorial services are prime moments out of time for reflection, adjustments, daily conversation, repentances, and apologies. They are personal and societal opportunities for positive realignment, based on solid renewal possibilities, and aspirations based on personal trust, compassion, and good will. These opportunities should be viewed as pure gold. An internal posture of compassion, trust, and goodwill toward oneself can be renewed, rebuilt, and shared through family, friend, job, and social functions. We are our ancestors. As the elders of the Hopi Tribe of Arizona say in their commentary and prophesy of current and future times, "We are the ones we have been waiting for."

These occasions can be posted within a drawn structure representing the Medicine Wheel. How is the Wheel drawing coming along?

When we arose out of the Divine Mind, differentiated into the world of duality, and took physical form we began to desire things to do and we deeply wanted to understand. The Medicine Wheel, the natural world, and we ourselves are the notes to be posted for things to do and ways by which to understand or begin to understand.

Let us lay down some flowers or put down some tobacco offerings at the altars of our own conception. With these offerings, so, too, do the perceptions of separation with the Creator have a chance to narrow, heal, and close in wholeness and trust and, so, too, can personal trust grow. And as extensions of this trust grows, our being as the Sacred Flowering Tree flourishes, growing deep, high, and wide, capable of recognizing, accepting, and supporting all manner of diverse life...for indeed, all life is diverse. In diversity is found our unique beauties and unities.

In daily life we interface, depend upon, and make use of everything, often without ceremony, offering, seeking permission, acknowledgement or gratitude, or even notice. Most things are freely given, but often we remain unceremonious takers. It is these unconscious actions that silently collect around our spirits and silt in around deeply unconscious needs to fulfill the ancient give and take (receive) premises upon which our world was conceived. This further erodes unconscious feelings of personal and collective trust, contributing further to feelings of unworthiness and disconnect with the Creator. Each person then disassociates, projects, or internalizes these feelings in an attempt to reason, understand, and manage mysterious separation anxieties, making us prey to those aforementioned ancient and unknown forces, spirits, or energies, benign or not, with which we coexist on the Mother Earth.

The history of the cosmos and of our Mother Earth–Father Sky-Sun contains many epochal layers, pages and chapters. Most of these chapters, if not blessed or resolved, ritually released and returned to Spirit, reside at other levels of existence, most of which have nothing to do with us but occasionally we "bump into" them, only becoming aware of them when a tear in the separating veil through accident, travel, chance or trauma, the media or possibly through simple misadventure brings contact. Meeting with one of these unfamiliar energetic collections is one of the prime reasons to hold postures of gratitude, engage in personal ceremony, collective prayer, purification and renewal activities such as, specifically, sweat lodges, fasting and purification fires, and the use of the sacred herbs for clearing, blessing, and holding firm, the most high, light, and grounded of positive atmospheres.

If one *does* perchance come into contact with "iffy," real or perceived negative energies, know that there is a life lesson here, waiting for a transformative meeting of a lifetime. What to do?

Remember first of all that you are a sacred being of God and *never, ever* forget it. And when it is forgotten, which it will be, remember, fan off, or think it, with the sacred herbs, and go on. Then immediately endeavor to remember all of the proven and worthy tools which you have been given, heard of, told, or can think of, and begin to enact those teachings closest and most available, such as asking the sage beings to help out and dispel negative energies. Petition the cedar beings to bring their positive and loving energies and, lastly, evoke the sweetgrass beings to fill any spaces that have been voided of fear, sorrow, anger, and judgment, leaving vulnerable and open spaces, possibly feeling abandoned, to be filled with love until *you* choose with what to refill those spaces. Emptied spaces can represent holes that may be attractive to roaming opportunistic entities. Make sure they are filled with the gifted smoke of plant love and your own gratitude.

The tests of faith come more often than we would like and are common to all. When they are not willingly and successfully met, deep feelings of unworthiness, entitlement, or mistrust arise and are internalized or projected. This, then, becomes one of the principle blocks toward maintaining vibrant connection with the Creator. When the tests, unattractive and distressful as they may be, are fully met with your medicine bundle of innate faith, gratitude, and fire ceremonies, personal trust in oneself, and the knowledge that one *will* and *can* survive and flourish beyond the possible death-dealing situations, then trust will be rebuilt.

The core energetic of loss of trust lies in the fact that as takers of life we begin to harbor deep suspicions that we are not life givers but are instead, simple takers and possibly killers. For the seeds that have so easily given themselves to us that have not been merged with and been given new life through continuing life with us, are instead gone. Now, we all know that nothing can ever really be killed, only transitioned, so rest a little easier. But when we let down our end of the give and receive contract of life, we may come to a very uncomfortable, unhealed, and unrestored position regarding our food, breath, water, and fire allies. Meanwhile, the deepest tests are designed to bring us to the recognition of fears that we may indeed be the killers. *Ouch!* And so, by the Ways of the Holy World and with the help of the Creator, our desperation, the memory of our spirit helpers and Ways, our prayers and the purification fires, this point can be successfully met and satisfied.

The basic failures of trust in ourselves and others can and will be healed. An event of this large and drastic a nature may never be yours to meet. However, if it does happen to you or a loved one, you will now be better informed and prepared, so you can make explanations to the best of your ability, allay paralyzing fears of imminent death confidently, and better know what steps to take. You will be in a better position to stabilize yourself or another person.

Begin by building a serious purification fire, in the purification fire mode, and feed it with tobacco offerings, prayers, and gratitude. Do these things on a cookie sheet inside the house if necessary. As soon as possible, proceed to "fan off" the affected party with the dry sacred herbs. A medicine event of this nature and magnitude will be accomplished quickly, so quickly as to be almost unbelievable, and will be accompanied by immediate feelings of and the knowledge of balance, harmony, and trust being restored. Trust that an action can not, and will not, take a long time. You or the treated person will be shaken up and should eat, drink water, and rest for some time. Integration will take some days. Continue fanning off and do not dwell on the difficulties, but immediately begin a renewed commitment to the mental and heartfelt discipline of the Gratitude Principle Teachings.

Monumental events of this nature, when experienced alone or witnessed by bystanders, can and perhaps will be diagnosed and viewed as a serious breakdown or episode when they may be or are, in point of fact, creative Medicine opportunities to make vast gains in restoring Spirit connection. It is through rough initiations of this nature that the last and largest impediments to restorations of balance, harmony, and connection to self and the Creator are realized…forever. These things often only happen once in a lifetime. Once personal trust and connection is healthy and in place, one will be seen as, and more importantly felt to be, a trustworthy person and will view others as more trustworthy. Balance and harmony is, or is on the Way to, being restored. A serious lesson has been offered and learned from what may have been, or was seen to be, an extremely negative or even dangerous condition arising out of a mysterious or invisible trans-plane history of existence. Perhaps these things are not intrinsically negative, but contact with them may be hard. The potential here is the lesson on trust. Once an encounter of this kind is accomplished, give thanks, go forward with a heart full of gratitude, and think on it no more. A renewal has taken place. Live gratefully and mindfully in the present with love and compassion for yourself and all living beings. *Aho!*

However, if an action of this sort results in extended psychosis or someone presents a physical danger to themselves and others, please do seek medical assistance immediately!

It is our sacred charge to live well, be happy, and to recognize ourselves as co-Creators, and either we *are* mindfully doing so or we are *not* doing this. Most of humanity is highly empowered and views itself as so highly entitled that it feels life is ours to pick and choose from, almost completely overlooking the serious work of daily and dedicated memory, disciplined thought, and the eternal application of the basic creative and gratitude principles by which our beautiful world was created and is still created. It is our prayers that keep our world going.

And now, I absolutely have to go receive the renewal medicine of a bowl of beans, chili, salt, and corn.

June 3, 2014, 9:26 CST

Another Dawn @ the Ranch

Wild Roses and Santa Rosa Plums

The heat of summer ripens and matures the swelling milkweed pod of the field, causes the green corn to dance, the sacred blackberry, *mkedémen,* to sweeten, the mountain lion to press deep tracks in damp clay, the mullein spikes to bloom yellow medicine for the mind, the bullfrog to bellow, and the nighthawk to sound. Small birds chase impossibly big birds from the nesting areas, tiny things emerge to sing their song and dance their dances.

Summer always offered the best possibilities to my father when, as a very young child and semi-orphaned, he often depended upon the kindnesses of strangers, lived in caves, and looked for wild food. The food he found most often was the wild plum. Since the plum bushes grew freely by roadways and creeks, no one laid claim to them or saw him as taking property that was not his to take.

Later, when he was grown and taking the family on road and camping trips he would always emerge from a grocery store with sardines, bread, bologna, mayo, some candy bars, and a sack of plums. It didn't matter what kind they were or even if they were ripe and sweet, which they seldom were, he would heft one, turning it in his hand like it was pure gold and he had food! I ate a lot of sour-cored plums.

This year two Santa Rosa semidwarf plum trees are planted in the garden to commemorate wild food.

June 16, 2014, 16:29 CST

Picking and Gathering for Balanced Health and Well-Being

Picking and gathering activities are most active in the summer and fall. Most or all plants have an optimum time of the month, their placement in the growth cycle, and specific areas of the plant for given application to specific conditions. The plant parts may be flower, pollen, seed, stem, leaf, or root. In the old Indian way many plants had specific songs, which were handed down, learned by example, or taught to individuals seen to exhibit that or those particular medicines. In these songs you would call the name of the plant, introduce yourself, and explain why they were being called to "help out." The songs were honoring and permission-seeking ways that grew out of close personal experience and relationship. Many of these ways have gone through a lot of changes, and it is now up to us to divine the fresh and new name-calling and honoring songs. This is a large part of the natural selection and personal-choice fulcrum upon which turn many of the Ways by which we participate in writing the new calendars, books of days, and positive evolutions while yet in a body cradled by the Medicine Wheel Web of Life, the

Mother Earth, the Father Sky-Sun, the Grandmother Moon and star people, helper Spirits, elementals, and ancestors—arisen afresh with each dawn of a new day, vibrantly emanating from the mind, heart, body, and spirit of the Creator and the Seed Beings who have produced babies.

Plant talks: Plant talks lead to the little marriages, which are a direct outgrowth of the winter prayer talks and songs initiated in the winter when the seeds of inspiration were fired. Whether or not we planted the particular seeds which resulted in the medicine seed and plant discussed here is known only to the farmer or gardener. The mullein plant described is naturalized in my garden and liberally shared with anyone who is interested.

SPIRIT TALK

The mullein plant being first spoke to me many years ago and has been a good friend and beautiful companion to myself and others over the years. It is a personal medicine that I now feel it time to broadly share. This medicine understanding and connection was not passed to me by anyone else, and so I will not offend a giver, friend, or teacher who also moves in a direct line of connection with the mullein beings and has anything to say about this decision. This is between myself, the Creator, the mullein beings, and you. You, I give the gift to in the name of humanity, unencumbered by ties of ownership or suggestions of if, how, to whom, and why you might be moved by Spirit and share this information. My uncle Bear Heart and other high teachers have taught me that the time for secrets is over. Humanity has too much need for information sharing to occupy proprietary positions where health, well-being, fellowship, compassion, and a continued positive evolutionary track is to be built, held, and followed. That being said, certain deeply held medicines will be very judiciously and selectively handled. This policy is also open for your consideration. When in doubt remember to ask, "Spirit, what's going on here?" That way we don't slant the answer because, after all, we don't know the answer or we wouldn't be asking, would we? Endeavor to be open to new information, follow up with another question for clarification, and then be prepared to follow your heart or intuitive connection to universal wisdom and make a personal choice. In these Ways do personal medicines emerge, strengthen, build, and grow.

More Marriage Talks: The Mullien plant spoke to me while on a return car trip from a high summer ceremony. It was one of those medicine drives where my husband and I pulled off the road every few miles, taking hours to cover ninety miles or so. We were in balance and harmony with the day. At one pull-off point lived many blooming mullein beings. Now, it is universally known that when the broad leaf is picked "in a good way" it is a healing aid to sprains, bruises, dislocations, and bone breaks, so I took this opportunity to gather a few leaves. Many women I know keep a paper sack of dried mullein leaf put by for such uses. For use, the leaf is moistened by water and the addition of some of your prayerful spit and breath, and either broken up or used whole and wrapped around the hurting and broken spot, then wrapped close but not tight with a cloth and tied securely. The spit, a sacred body fluid, carries the healing prayer to the mullein being, partners with it, and begins to restore order and harmony where it has been compromised. Unwrap, wash the area when it seems right, and reapply unless the child is already up, off the sofa, and playing outside. Deeper or more intense sprains will take overnight or longer. (NOTE: I caution you though, do not hesitate to take the injured person for an X-ray or doctor's attention if the injury is very painful, sharp, or long lasting. Never keep anyone away from the emergency room if they are asking for it or appear to need skilled assistance.) Then, gather up the particles, go outside, return the medicine to the Mother and "put down" some tobacco in gratitude for the life and health restoring gifts lent by the mullein beings.

The Broken Ground

Mullein grows on broken ground. This is its medicine. The specific medicine I was given on the "long medicine drive" day went like this. Remember, it is a beautiful day. I am feeling connected in a balanced and harmonious way with Creation…being positively sensitized with the day, the plants, and yourself is the most important part of this teaching. Overriding or overlooking this necessary condition will have its own teaching to impart,…and so your story and medicine understanding will progress.

Personal harmony is the authentic spirit ground from which the medicine conversations are conducted. To initiate this medicine relationship, wait or watch for a time of deeply experienced personal connection with the natural world and yourself to conduct the first gathering. There are more observances and suggestions regarding picking and gathering to be found in the Autumn segment of this book, so I suggest skimming forward and adding this material to your thoughts and preparations. Now let's say a time has been identified, perhaps unexpectedly. If you are feeling interested and attended to this information, I suggest you secure a bit of offering tobacco and carry it about your person in order to be prepared at all times for a divinely offered opportunity to gather a medicine plant of interest, whether it be mullein or another plant.

We are now deep within the Medicine Wheel Teachings and no longer know it. I am at the roadside gathering mullein leaves and come to know it would be a good thing to gather some of the yellow (summer color) flowers growing on the long spike tips. I am listening and obeying. I ask some of the flowers to come with me and help out…the pick goes easily as I insert a thumbnail, no metal, at the flower base and put it safely away until the "enough" message is received.

I take the flowers home and spread them out to dry on a cloth or paper, and while I am within that process more information comes in the form of a "knowing" that a tea made with these flowers would bring a calm and healing sleep to a mind temporarily "broken" by a traumatic event. I steeped and drank some tea for myself in preparation, and soon a situation presented itself where the tea was mindfully brewed and restored order and harmony within a restful sleep to a mind temporarily disturbed by a family loss, disappointment, or other trauma.

SPIRIT TALK

Handle the dried mullein flowers as you would pieces of yourself. Greet them, introduce yourself again, remember and relive the day when you came together. It was a good day, a very, very good day.

Gently lower the blossoms into the simmering water, cover the pan (glass is best, if at all possible), remove from the heat and steep for fifteen to twenty minutes. Pour, cool, and give one teacup of the tea to the distraught person, then see that they can lie down and go to sleep. See that they drink all of the tea. Any extra can be refrigerated but try not to make more than one cup at a time. No more will be needed. Drink it yourself as an honoring if there is extra. Return the flowers to the Mother with gratitude and put down some tobacco as a culturally recognized offering. You may diverge in this offering in the future, as guided, but for now this tobacco is a universally recognized currency on Turtle Island, America, Sweet Medicine land. The other currency, and the only real one, is the balanced and harmonious heart. This is what the spirit of the Mullein Being recognizes and consents to partner and work with...balance and harmony, ours and theirs, that is the working and active element of the medicine.

The yellow-flower sleep will then transport the distressed sleeper to the time and place of the gather, the day, the season, the breezes, mists, clouds, hummingbirds, and the ants which are always found to be climbing the spikes. These are the things which make "good medicine." This is why it is important to pick in a good way. This is who we are and what we have to offer. This also goes for song, thoughts, actions, the written and spoken word. It is never not right.

Other Gifts of the Mullein Beings: While I have only heard of this use and do not have actual experience I will put it forward for treatment of those with "broken" lungs. The smoke of the dry mullein leaf is medically recognized to have a demulcent effect on the lungs when lightly breathed, which could be helpful with conditions like emphysema. Proceed with caution. I suggest breathing a bit of the smoke if you are considering applying this remedy personally in order to have firsthand experience, and then always be in attendance when asking the medicine if it will "help out" and offering the tea.

In conclusion, Spirit Talks, marriage talks, and prayers are *always* to be done as far in advance as possible. This practice, should it speak to you, will change your life. I seemed to notice that Uncle did not go into and out of prayer, he was always in some state of prayerful gratitude, play, laughter, appreciation or ceremony. He was fun to be around. "Be happy," he would say, "there is so much beauty around, wake up!"

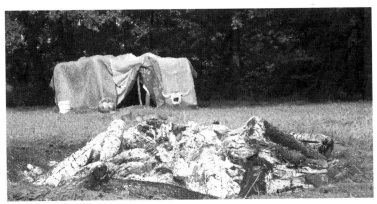

The Sweat Lodge

June 21, 2014

THE SUMMER SOLSTICE

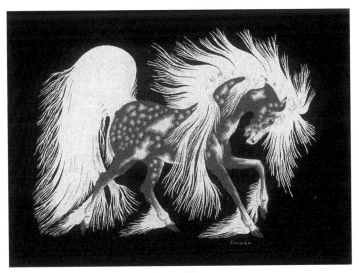

Spirit Horse

If we don't "go over" to the teachings of the natural world we're missing a prime evolutionary moment, for the human species is no longer in the ascendancy. Our projected paths have both narrowed precipitously and broadened radiantly. The choice is ours...actually there probably *is* no choice about whether we will successfully evolve in harmonious concert with the Mother Earth, only about the individual degree of personal choice one forms and occupies regarding participation.

June 16, 2014, 24:00 CST

The Summer Marriage Talks

The marriage talks have begun in earnest and the couplings are begun. All witnesses are gathered and attendants clustered around the sacred circles. Everywhere! Sacred circles are everywhere. There's one, and there...and there! It's all sacred circles, a never ending, endless swarming and swelling sea of warm and wet sacred circles. Circles, which have arisen full blown from the conscious prayer, song, hope, and dream...Circles manifesting at last, out of the winter high seed ceremonies. High seed circles arising from our familiar dream, but mostly, circles that have arisen unknown, new and unbidden by ourselves from bird droppings, raccoon scat, coyote vomited peach pits, clouds of wind carried pollen, diffused mushroom spore, gravel beds of salmon egg and sperm in a fog of milt...Circles mothered and fathered out of the vast and unfathomable creative recesses and pinnacles of the Creative Mind whose fingers, veins, loamy composts, and pervasive warmths not only host the dreamed circles but extend bountiful permissions to initiate and support tomorrow's fresh and unique flowering trees and flying fish.

The marriage talks arrive with us. With summer and the solstice we make ready to accept the unknown, and make ourselves ready, adorned in our resplendent fullness and beauty to process down the great seasonal aisle and make the marriage with *ourselves* first of all! When we moved into the great dream and experiment of the duality principle, the perception of separation from the Creator became the first wound, and out of that wound came the life blood of our essential heartbeat's desire to close that perceived and achingly real gap with the Creator. Duality became the physical and actual metaphor for our sense of inner separation and personal creativity—a driving evolutionary force toward the ultimate goal of *unifying* those exceptionally beautiful and diverse aspects of differentiation, the assignment of gender roles.

The marriage talks are all about the merging of gender roles toward the attainment of unity, beyond gender parity, encompassing and incorporating as never before, an ultimate vision, the reach and grasp of promised co-creativity. The co-creativity that has been written and spoken of, dreamed and envisioned, sensed and longed for, initiated into, and finally, most often, undelivered but by physical transition. We occupy now, an unprecedented opportunity to merge with the promised co-creative powers while still in the body. Many and strange will be the paths toward making this push forward beyond what we have known or been able to accomplish, and the most secure and historically known format by which to initiate ourselves beyond the comfortable and known is still the sacred Medicine Wheel, the directions, colors, seasons, and center core of unity, where the Sacred Tree of Life flowers and all of our circuitous paths merge with the ever renewing fertile flower of possibility.

The Sacred Circle as the Wedding Ring

The first aisle walked is our own, the consenting marriage of differentiation. Ah, yes, we must look across the divide and aisle at our other, be it male or female, and be willing to see beyond difference. We must be willing to see the beauty of our other half, the severed half of our Sacred Flowering Tree and if we be willing to take another chance, agree to join and make the walk toward blessed soul unity. What that looks like we won't know. And it won't be the only time we will make the talks and take the walks,…but there will be more, many, many more, and trust that they will become easier and more comfortable as new flowering coats are assumed and relinquished with the seasons. Courage, endurance, and bravery be ours, always.

The Sacred Staff as the Aisle

The sacred staff, our spine, forms what is called the Good Red Road. You will remember that Good Red Road connects the northern white, spirit breath of winter purity with the southern red, heart-felt emotion of summer love. This walk is a good one... They are all good but this one is key for it provides valuable and obvious keys of discerning practicality regarding the observance and evaluation of the choices, activities, the givens and gifts arising out of the all-important "Firing the Seeds of Inspiration" of winter, which began our new year, and observing the practical and visibly manifested outcomes of that effort and partnership with the Mother Earth, Father Sky-Sun and the Holy Mind of the Creator, as the powers of the north and south marry and show of what they are made...and more.

The Marriage Attendants and the Wedding Gifts

The marriage attendants are the *everything*. We will never know the actual fullness of the knowingness. The wedding gift is us, and the resultant fullness of those trusting steps taken toward inner healing, wholeness, beauty, and unity is a core reality platform from which to dare to dream, build, and experience a holy and sacred Earth walk, a walk which we can now safely consider to be entering into the marriage talks with another sacred circle.

The wedding gifts are us, an unreserved outflow of abundant medicine accrued giveaway bounty in gratitude for being given the sacred gift of life—our payback, if you will, for being allowed to work, serve, suffer, to love and to be loved whilst within the dream of life.

The Dream of Life

The dream of life is our ephemeral experience, one where we emerge out of unity, recognize and build personal and common values, live a certain individuality within the inner and outer collective dream, and at certain other incremental points, evolve and eventually merge once more into complete unity, the Spirit from whence we originated…a larger marriage.

The Good Red Road Is Built

The Good Red Road has been built and accomplished for this year. It always has been and, now, will always be a strong, straight, and true alignment and reference point for the infallible inner compass, our compass true and trusted.

The Hard Road of Life

The hard road of life is under construction, well under construction, and will be open for travel in the fall. The hard road of life— our arms—connect the east: spring, fire, yellow, mental, direction of illumination and inspiration, with the direction of the west: autumn, water, physical, black or dark blue color, with the medicine attributes of introspection. When the mind marries with the physical it is called the hard road of life but always, it meets and crosses with the Good Red Road of heart, where they meet the sacred tree flowers.

The Sacred Flowering Tree

The Sacred Flowering Tree is every person's sacred gift and manifestation, always freshly arising out of and into its own Sacred Circle and engaged in never ending marriage talks with God and self. Our relationship to ourselves is about the same as our relationships to others, common creative values connecting our creativity to the Creator, the Great Mystery, and the gifts that rise out of duality: the Natural World.

The Personal Wedding

Personal ceremony for oneself can be considered and celebrated anytime, but this season is rotund with possibility and opportunities for giveaway. One can be both the bride and groom, neither spirit being given-away, owned, bought or stolen, nor taking-on, but moving forward with joint consent into the two-made-one, true marriage of and into unity with self within the Great Mystery.

> *Dream, Dance, Feast, Giveaway!*
> *Laugh, Love, and Be Happy!*
> *Sleep, Heal, Forgive, Repent!*
> *Cry, Renew, Die and be Reborn*

Be a Great Summer Ceremony...*Being is doing...*

Or, draw a Sacred Circle of like-minded beings near and design an honoring and celebrating High Summer Solstice Ceremony, where the winter prayer seed meets the summer seed dressed in all of its finery,...and then...

Play the parts, tell the stories, remember.

Be the falling rain or snow, be the warm or frozen Mother Earth, be the shorter or longer rays of Father Sky-Sun. Be the unfurling shoot, be the yellow leaf of fall.

Dance the world alive with the strong, cold male rains and the soft, walking female rains.

Make the roll call of sentient beings with the special spring bird song

THE GREAT SUMMER CEREMONIES

The great summer ceremonies, no matter what seed; tribe; culture; fur, skin, fin, scale, or feather; code, nation, ancestral, initiatory, religion, or collective consciousness are always and ever an honoring marriage of all seeded beings, warm and cold bloods, and the two-legged heart as each dances with the Creator...a giveaway that life can go on "in a good way." Dream and make fresh, vibrant, and new ceremonies arising out of personal medicine that tradition might continue to move hand in hand, heart in heart with the Creator and all living things, now and forever more. *Aho!*

The Summer Marriages

No sooner are the summer marriages made and new seeds on the way, staged to begin broadcasting new and old genetic memory, than the steep changes of autumn appear in the distance as small, pale medicine mountains. Soon they will appear to rise out of the ground, darkening in color, bearing promise of sweet and bitter harvest, cool evergreen forests, rushing mountain streams and sheer rocky cliffs; hot July nights and drying southern winds, monsoon rains and red tides. The way to the medicine mountains is still over and across the white plain, now sere and dry but incredibly beautiful when one gets down on the stomach for a mouse eye view. It's another world, previously unknown and underfoot. It distracts and pacifies us for a while from thinking about the slow and inexorable advance of this new great mystery, autumn.

As the human umbilicus presses against the elemental Mother body, she says softly, "Look here, look here," meaning the white plain and what lies beneath, as if speaking to an overactive, tired, and distracted young one running about, drunk on life.

The last twenty-one days of summer reds and greens become more deeply tinted, as the autumn blacks sit in their place of the west, medicine direction, to receive and introspect summer's seed, initiating the closing journey with the winter whites of purity and wisdom.

A new creation story is being made, coming forward for winter telling and to prepare us for the new year with tales of a well-known path meant to tell beauty, dispatch qualms, questions, and fears of the new and unknown. The new stories are being made on every given breath. Pay attention to every little thing, be grateful, and accept life in whatever form it is encountered and lived.

Summer—the Twenty-one Days Before Autumn Begins

The Autumnal Twilights Commence and the Thirteen Blue Corn Moons Measure Time

The night after the Capricorn Full Moon is velvety black and silent. The moon casts the weakest of shadows and illuminates nothing beneath the trees, and the following morning is still and quiet. The summer Sun begins to move us into the edges of all twilight. The summer Sun leads us forward into the autumn by softening the fiery mental resolves and physical intentions, by sponsoring the moist marriage heart's urge to seed and all the while, the Sun Spirit slowly continues winding the cyclical fibers of being upon the spool of spiral time, drawing us forward, binding the drying stalks and fruits into sheaves of harvest.

Already, seed imprints know themselves. Knowledge of ourselves stumbles and looks about for clue and information. Most seeds remain encased in tender and tough sheaths until the final days of "making" are complete. The twilight presages the deep rest, sleep, and quiet time but for now, calm and caution, softening and waiting are the appropriate stances. These things, all things, ourselves, require this time, time to draw and color what has been "made." It is our time to "make" the imaginary Spirit drawings and color in the first sketches out of the water filled ollas of summer. The winter stories, songs, and dances continue to form and flesh out, gaining momentum in contrast to the outward-looking stillnesses. It remains too soon to speak of the stories, to sing the song which is still but a hum, and to dance what is still a walk, but we are coming to know some things, and also know there is much more to come.

The late summer rains are fewer. The mulching, irrigation, and sprinkling the rows of tasseling corn, which is gaining its majority, is required, so too directed water streams are flowing down the thirsty rows and gullets of growth. Clouds of pollen drift down upon the fair hairy heads of slim corn bodies. The final "making" is done in the dry heat.

The passages upon the thirteen-moon calendar continues in beauty...

July 23, 2014 9:32:25 AM

Our Seed Emerges with the First Harvest

Be alert, aware, and look within during the first four days of the new season, for our new seeds will begin to make themselves known. The academic or curious path from the new year seed firing ceremonies in December will begin to bear a personal seed harvest. We *are* the fields we have been tending and the new seeds are freshly arisen from within the quarters of wisdom and purity; inspiration and illumination; love and trust; and now they begin to make the mysterious marriage with introspection and medicine. The violet twilight path into the autumnal "crack between the worlds" is relating to the daily evening "crack between the worlds" we experience regularly. So pace yourself to welcome the familiar, but now it is upon the larger calendar of the thirteen moons. If a drawing of "days" is being followed, identify your placement and enter it with sound, color, animal, plant, and directional orientation.

July 23, 2014 9:47:50 AM

AUTUMN, SEED

Do you recall the first words of this writing and how they arose from within and out of the first four days of Quiet Time, when the Mother rests? Consider then, viewing this fourth and final initiation into the fourth and final quarter of the Medicine Wheel to be similar in sacred nature. Set aside these four days for special observation of your own making. Be calm, quiet and mindful as possible, vigilant of gifts, inspiration or idea, and especially of the support of others which may have quietly grown up around us since December. All of these things are seed food. Seed food appearances are giveaway times so prepare to giveaway in recognition and celebration of the new seeds that have arisen out of an essential state of being, which has elected to move within and alongside of the Sacred Medicine Wheel of the Mother Earth and the Father Sky-Sun.

But before thoughts of the giveaway bounty goes any further, let us pause for one very long moment, perhaps a lifetime, to recognize, appreciate and seat this precious seed newcomer, securely in the center of our being. All that we need and are, for the one being, is within us. We have drawn of the powers, been given-away to by the powers of Creation and are made anew! This then, is what life is about at its best. It is time to observe big, inner ceremony.

Such seed neither seeks nor has need of external validation. This is valuable.

This seed knows itself to be a complete and discrete, self-capable of knowing and reproducing itself and knowing the seed essences of others.

SPIRIT TALK

We are the new seed…brought forward from the old stock and tended until the new crop is produced. Sit with and within this complete seed. Come to know the completeness *it* sits within, for it has reproduced itself and grown to meet, mutate, adjust to, and incorporate the new earthly conditions and prayer contributions it has met. Now, make a thoughtful and willing merge with your new seed self. This new seed self is here, now, because it is an inseparably connected particle of Creation and *also* because it is a freestanding and individuated particle of Creation. It represents a definition of wholeness, balance, and harmony at its best. Accept and draw in whatever aspect of this gift is most apparent and available this moment. Draw it in deeply. Allow it to merge with and nourish and renew every cell history and its potential; every memory of muscle, blood, bone, and mind; every emotion and emotional patterning; every externalized need, desire, and envy; every misuse of power ever turned upon us, known or unknown, and every misuse of power wielded by us; allow it to mend or begin to mend every suffering moment arising out of fear, sorrow, anger, judgment, chemical imbalance, or visited negative influence of any kind,…now and forever more.

This is one of the major Ways by which we keep our world going "in a good way." Sit with this earned and worked for gift long and hard. Never let it go and never forget it. Watch it grow, co-Creator! This is a sacred moment of all sacred moments. This moment has been dreamed of, prayed for, cried and agonized over; read of, hoped for, and heard of, cynically forgotten and then—out of a survival mode—disbelieved, distanced from, and yet seen and remembered in every rainbow and young thing. When these mixed conditions of life have been met, recognized, accepted, and walked, and the paths and truths have been taken to and within the Medicine Wheel full-life experience, then our pictures and understandings can mature and come to, or begin coming to, fruition in a comprehensive and orderly fashion.

Out of this mixed bounty, arise the future conditions necessary for successive growth, and it is from the deep, profoundly purified and renewed inner seed sprouts that the initial (initiated) concepts, impulses, and urges for sharing and the giveaway mind is formed. The simple giveaways of the talking circles, recipes for food, advice and teachings, voices raised in song, dance, chant and prayer, art and utility crafts, labor, nursing and doctoring... all of the earthly tendings, and love, respect, and honoring ways all grow from this bounty.

The spring and autumnal twilights bring a special power, beauty, and potential to the Medicine Wheel year. They are the worked for and grown arms of the east-west axis of the spring emergence and the west point of completion, balance, and harmony, which serve and fulfill the Unity center. These elementals are always working side by side—the north-south axis of the winter point of origin and the south point of abundant making and manifestation of the material plane.

We are completing this cycle.

We are now the New Seed, observing and celebrating the known and unknown mysteries, proceeding from the autumnal twilights ever more deeply into the deepest blue blacks of the deepest medicine of the introspective west to know the medicine mystery of completion, the mother of origin, and then,...to arrive, rest, and sleep in our Mother Earth's white winter nest of all return and birth awaiting the new seed firing ceremonies as she meets and makes Spirit Union with the fires of our Father Sky-Sun.

This year's journey is now complete. Welcome home journeyer and seeker of life's most profound instructions. We are now in a personal center of origin whereby we sought the original instructions on how to best be ourselves, to truly know all others, and to be a real human being.

For if the Creator God ever spoke to us, the speaking continues. And so it has and so it does, now and forever more. It is good. It is very, very good. *Aho!*

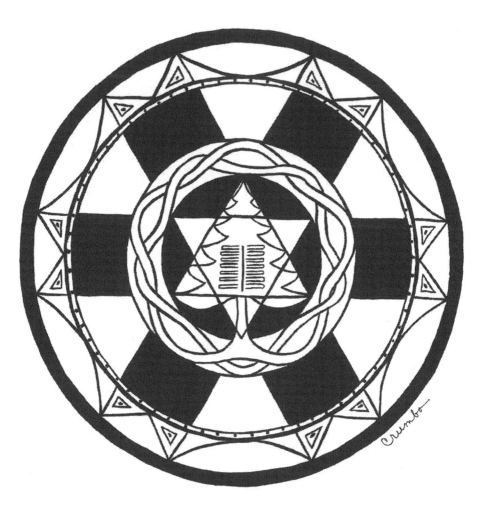

Tree of Life

The Tree of Life rests within ancient and ever-fresh symbols of celestial life, its roots sunk deep within the six-day creation cycle, the Whole representing the Seventh, day of rest.

Tree of Life
Minisa Crumbo

AUTUMN...DGWAGÉK

A new season arrives...

May it fire the seeds of inspiration, illumination, love, the medicine of introspection, wisdom, and purity as the winds and fires of Creation carry our spirits into and within the Spirit of peace and unity all the days of our lives, *forever...*

Migwech, Master of All Breath, *wewene kiche migwech*
Thank you, Creator, thank you very, very much

The Autumn Harvest and the Fall Equinox

The autumn harvest has a signature similar to all other completion and fulfillment moments, but is also uniquely different owing to its deep roots in the fundament of Creation. For this reason, it will always be counted as one of the original templates by which to gauge and measure natural progress of any kind. It mounts and takes its place as a real and conceptual template alongside the other seasons of winter, spring, and summer as a massive barometer and register that exceeds full comprehension. Autumn is a "crack between the worlds" of summer and winter and, as such, is similar to the crack between the worlds of spring, between winter and summer,…the dusks and dawns of the year. The sun stands still at the time of the autumn equinox, its light *balanced* by time, and becomes the physically visible *balance* beam, fourth quarter, of the Medicine Wheel.

The Path of Light

The western balance beam of the "hard road of life" completes, closes, and connects the western direction of medicine, introspection, and the physical with the eastern direction of inspiration, illumination, and the mental. The balanced path of light is our walk between body and mind, the path of the Sun as it traverses the sky and circulates in ceaseless mutual partnership and rhythm with the Earth. The path of light, the sunrises and sunsets, may be viewed as one half, an axis, of our lateral Earth walk, balance.

The other half of our Earth walk, the noons and midnights, may then be viewed as the cross beam of *harmony* that connects the southern direction of emotion, love, and the heart with the northern direction of purity, wisdom, and Spirit breath.

The connection center, where the Sacred Tree flowers and the World Tree grows, is a well-known and well-traveled crossroad upon the paths of balance and harmony, which connect both the outer and inner points on the Circle, a lunar, stellar, and solar system replication of our cosmos!

This diagram and seat of mind, heart, body, and Spirit energetics is encoded in everything. To understand this is to incorporate a comprehensive tool that can unlock the unknown by shining the intelligent light beams of balance and harmony, the center and unifying circle, in an identifying, receiving, and imprinting way upon all things. This structure is a metaphor for the intelligent mind, loving heart, creative and all-seeing eye, and adaptive body, stepping up to and inheriting a position as co-Creator in active evolution…most fully "alive in a loving world."

The words "balance" and "harmony" have oft been heard, repeated, spoken, written, sensed, hoped, and longed for. They may have been thought unattainable, at a distance, and then, as suddenly, the words can live and merge seamlessly with every fiber and quality of our being—blessing, encompassing, and affirming the inner framework of the Medicine Wheel and all that resides upon, within, or around it. The natural world personifies and exemplifies the merge of a center-unified balance and harmony, taking these qualities beyond emotional and mental concepts, making them visible, known, comprehensible, and available.

The natural world—the first, most beautiful and enduring of the Creator's gifts to us—will ever and always be our schoolhouse, lover, art gallery, Mother, Father, and Grandmother, friend, font of scientific discovery, teat, bloodier of knee and elbow, emergence point and final resting place...home. It is both a sanctuary and a mirror—a sanctuary where we can enter with nothing and simply be in Spirit and a mirror of our entire *beingness*, where we can also enter with all of our baggage and gifts. There is a place for everything and the void, in and on the Medicine Wheel.

The Summer Sun's Medicine Face of Love and Trust and the Summer Sun's Medicine Face of Fear and Mistrust

The active transit of this season presents the fulsome harvest opportunities to recognize and accept the bright shining faces of every new seed and then, when doing so, to lift and glide as high an eagle with the cosmic winds of Creation beneath our wings, bridging any and all perceived separation anxieties between or within ourselves, others, or the Creator.

The shadow face of the favorable and desirable summer sun is fear or mistrust. These two qualities travel with love and trust like night and day. They are the search and regeneration engines of the season. It is imperative that this is recognized and accepted as a facet of the Medicine Wheel pattern, which allows, accepts, and creates a nonjudgmental place for all things. Advance knowledge of this landscape can acknowledge high points of beauty, however growth and intra/interpersonal interactions can often be uneven, requiring that we employ the steadying directional arms of balance and harmony. The conscious and acknowledged presence of these arms, the east-west axis, incorporates and integrates evolving energetics in motion or transit—motions now steady, known, and balanced, now unsteady, unknown as to outcome, and momentarily out of balance,...like breath and the Earth walk.

As differing growth levels are encountered we may come to view even our own motives and actions with question, fear, or mistrust for they may smack of the unknown or different...the other. Thus, some core origins of fear and mistrust may arise to pass through the crucible of the Medicine Wheel and become the dross that is illuminated, refined, purified, transformed, and returned into the sound seed stock that was prayed over and inculcated with the conscious fires of inspiration and new life in December. We are the dreamers and the dreamed.

The Medicine Wheel, in all of its broad parameters, offers solid and stable strategies to meet the conditions and situations we may encounter, even the undesirable ones, for this is when and how we come to forge our authentic identities as co-creators. This is when, how, and why we do the work. Now, let us examine one of the most powerful shadow faces, fear and mistrust, to debunk and "doctor" them in the highest way possible in order that we might begin to put a end to all that is not true, close the gaps of real or perceived separations, and forge the shining faces of love and trust.

These great bugaboos of fear and mistrust, which often result in suspicion and jealousy, are very close in nature, a mirror face, to love and trust. They are treated and doctored similarly, even identically, with the proven and worthy tools of the Gratitude

Principle and Being Breathed. Let's go over some of the teaching again. The transformative tools of recognition, acceptance, and gratitude, when accompanied by the flushing and releasing activity of *expressing* gratitude, even before it can honestly be said to be experienced, is a primary tool. I here suggest revisiting the Gratitude Principle teachings. The restoration of order and harmony is essential and elemental. There really is no choice. If one desires to command self-respect and a measure of happiness this restoration of order must be taken seriously and seen to as quickly as possible. Once the Gratitude Principle is initiated, or reinitiated, you may fall back or forward into it with trust, as one does a habitual response, and observe its transformative power. One successful experience will provide all of the encouragement necessary to move forward.

The simple rebuilding of personal and interpersonal trust and love through acknowledging personal motivations first, taking nothing personally, and remembering to employ the proven and worthy tools until new habits and responses are formed can be relearned through willing and disciplined thought followed by constructive action. We might also consider the willingness and desirability or necessity to forgive ourselves or others, through understanding, sincere repentance, an appropriate and balanced restitution of some kind, an apology, or by asking someone if they can overlook a real or perceived offense while allowing everyone time to get over, or heal from, certain conditions, actions, or situations and to move on.

TRUSTING THE PROVEN AND WORTHY TOOLS

Suspicion, or the qualification of wholesome love and trust platforms, must not be allowed to taint or divide trust fields for long. Relevant questions, intuitions, feelings, information, and facts must be honored, examined, and perhaps held and inspected for a time for progress or conclusions to be reached by many means, but this is especially so through the introspective and substantive offices of the Medicine Wheel. Any suspicions, judgments, and jealousies exposed to the Medicine Wheel, or another selected system of ethical and moral conduct, will then have the best opportunities through purification and renewal to build not only foundations of true health, honor, love, and trust but also those of sound internal and external reasoning processes.

Remembering, retaining, and holding the proven and worthy tools are the necessary housekeeping implements to deal with specious issues and other, simply unfamiliar situations. As you grow in sensitivity and awareness, be prepared to meet and observe other, more mysterious and unknown qualities, such as visions, intuitions, and feelings perceived from ancient DNA, tribal, familial, karmic histories; songs or stories; spirit helpers from this or other realms; star people; directional energetics; dimensional bleed through; plants, winds, waters, or minerals communicating awareness and intelligence; and advanced studies from oral and written tradition. There will be much to learn and the most proven and worthy tools honed through use will allow you to entertain and examine new concepts and to discriminate trustingly, while temporarily suspending a familiar definition of known reality. There is positive growth potential here and there will be opportunities to refine further definitions of separation.

Separation and unification are the same things, defined by personal position, degree, and perception, through differing evolutionary vehicles. In reference to the Medicine Wheel, the experience of various stages, planes, and levels of individual evolution will call for, and allow for, the healthy and safe negotiation of mysterious avenues as the beautiful collective dream of duality translates into ever broader and equalized experiences. Transitions previously unknown to us, as we surfed the oceans of responsible attachment, will transform into and through seriously disquieting voids and vacuums as our attachment sensibilities, habits, affinities, compulsions, addictions, talents, and gifts undergo loosening and preparation exercises by which to lighten and clear the baggage, gifts, and proclivities of our lifetime(s) that grew out of the bounty of duality. These voids and vacuums may appear curiously, even alarmingly, empty and perhaps the teachings of the Spring white plain, appearing like chalk, will be recalled. These emptyings, voids, and vacuums are the clearing functions of a well-known way,…clearing and opening space for the brilliant and creative flow of life force and energy.

Surfing this dry white plain is best done by recognizing it as a transitional plain/plane were life force itself may appear to soften or ebb, as one enters into this creative void. A caution: during a serious transition of this type, even gratitude may be difficult to access, remember, or express, so fall forward or back as you prefer to view it, on your best and most highly formulated focus and related physical activity…Keep moving. The activity of holding a focus may be more important than the actual subject of the focus. This disciplined "tracking of the mind" will make an important contribution to holding positive equilibrium and the following restoration of normalcy.

These voids are designed to loosen and strip superfluous attachments to the historical desire body, opening energetic tunnels and reaming open new pathways of enhanced development and increased nourishment toward the evolution of Spirit. These can be spotty, difficult, although brief, passages. Be aware of these possibilities. While they may be mysterious and even hard, they are not intrinsically bad, unless you do something to harm yourself through diminished attention and trust.

That being said, there may be occasions when one may not be fully able to trust what they see or even think they know at these times. Proof and facts may appear to shift, disappear, or change form. This is a call to detach, wait, remain in focus, move, and await development of the larger picture. Endeavor to relate and define the information by placing it in an appropriate place on the Medicine Wheel by season, quality, or color. This will always be the initial step for evaluating information and making some sense of any question. Trust ultimately in the larger process of enhanced Soul development...Merge and fuse with the energies of the Creator, the Master of All Breath.

But then, just suppose that said question or suspicion is well-founded, grounded, or confirmed. These surviving perceptions of separation, if not checked, can create conditions fertile for the growth of additional disarray, arising from something as simple as a basic choice or difference. All I can say without going into "doctoring" specifics is this: The daily ceremonies will keep the blessing shields strongly activated in the auric field, and the innermost being will be most able and willing to exude balance and harmony to all who enter into said energy field, be that entry by thought, word, deed, Internet, or telephone. No shame, no blame. We will exude restoration of harmony and balance for anything or anyone that crosses into, or endeavors to penetrate, our energy field uninvited, by whatever means. That penetration, at our core source, comes only for a blessing! Including blessings to ourselves, right? Nothing is hurt and all things benefit by having a little love sent that way.

SPIRIT TALK

It is better to be part of the solution instead of part of the problem. Choice is a sacred right. Utilize it and take the road less traveled,...the Good Red Road that connects heart with Spirit and the Hard Road of Life that connects mind with body,...and rest always in the center where the Sacred Tree flowers.

THE VIOLET TWILIGHT
OF AUTUMNAL INGRESS REVISITED

A twilight beam may accompany the white plain as we progress into the western arm of medicine and introspection. Even as the light may seem to dim and take on a violet cast, the inner vision grows stronger and fundamental structures and building blocks are sketched dim now, now stronger...And faith, trust, and knowledge grow new legs, eyes, and ears, as we progress toward the deepest inner fires of December, winter, and the New Year. The light clears of core-fire blue violet and swells to join the orange flames and fires to which the historic and new seed faces are brought to experience a return and renewal at the inner-fire sources of purification and inspiration.

The winter fire-womb of the year approaches and deep within, the body of the Mother has received the penetrating shafts of heating, generating, and illuminating fires both from the inner earth core of the Mother and from the outer Father Sky-Sun. That is where we are inexorably headed as we transit this season, into the womb for the firing of the seeds with vision and the breath of life necessary to make life again, next year. Different cultures assign gender roles to these principles based on experience, vision, and tradition. Yours may differ but in the end, the fires are the powers by which we live,...by whichever name they are called. The fire beings are the Sacred and Holy gifts to us from Prime Creator, the Master of All Breath.

Take heart, be courageous, brave, faithful, and loving. Be prepared to endure that which must be endured and prepared to receive the gifts along the way and to never, ever, forget that we are Sacred Beings. From the Divine we originated and to the Divine we shall return,...and all the way through! The new paths will soon become clearer. The new and strengthening tools of our knowingness—prehensile eyes, ears, and senses—will develop and grow as required, naturally and undramatically. Anticipate change and evolution to gently and normally unfurl fresh opportunities and expanding powers of comprehension as vital new paths are observed, chosen or not, and walked. Greet them and offer welcome, and join through the new paths of unified potential with our first, elemental parents, the Mother Earth and the Father Sky-Sun, and know life.

Finally, it is wise to consider doing a perceptional sweep of separation signals. When signals are found to be lingering, hidden, camouflaged, latent, or obviously personal or observed, they are but steady and usually reliable responses to the annual energetic shifts of previous seasons—the highly energetic summer growth patterns, last growth, and early harvest. This journey into the deeper waters, fires, ethers, winds, stones, *skebyak*, and bodies of autumn is trustworthy and desirable. Cast about for the highest intentions and select one or some for focus. Prepare to hold this ground, moving forward with breath and the seasonal impulses until the firmer autumnal ground can be felt beneath your feet. This seasonal transit is the final one before the return. It represents potent approaches and transitions through the boundaries of the qualities of the physical, medicine, and introspection of the west. This is where, when, and how the power axis of of east-west, balance and harmony, join and take up their posts to complete and stabilize the north-south, Good Red Road, and join and the core of the Sacred Hoop. All *skebyak* (the green beings), the animal beings, two-leggeds, rock, water, fire, and wind beings know and go through these things.

The experience of linear time has many qualities...push-pull, vacuum, stasis. A full immersion into a life shared with the Medicine Wheel Teachings will also contribute to the place of the Eternal Present, where one is able to live fully in the moment and *be*. We, and all others, are on this journey. Smile, look about, rest, maintain, work, take care of the physical plant, help, love, and honor one another, meet the personal ceremonies of "being breathed," the Spirit Plate offerings, daily sunrise observances, all gratitude services. Allow these and other rituals to guide, recall, and support our willingness and enthusiasm by which to make a return to natural "good ways to live." These and other personal and collective daily ceremonies will provide and indicate irreplaceable and unparalleled direction and support, at times when none other will seem apparent, and offer sustenance when things are going well.

SPIRIT TALK

This way,…when all of the perceptions of separation are healed and rejoined and the time comes when we make ready to "lay down our bag of bones" we will be able to transition lightly into Spirit. And even if we do not have to lay down our bag of bones, our travel will be lighter. The absence of separation will be fulfilled with completion and fused with the knowledge of Unity with all living things. The diligence applied to this season prepares all things for the annual meetings of clearance and completion, resolving key and core separation-unity issues, thus easing us gently into the kindling emergence fires of wisdom, purity, and Spirit Breath…Winter.

This year's paths have been walked. We sit in a center of our universe and call it good. The harvest is being picked and gathered; cleaned and sorted; evaluated and counted, for we would remember, "every harvest is a new beginning," "every seed is counted as a new tomorrow."

Now is a good time to invite and organize a Circle gathering, going deep within the year, marking and celebrating the first harvests and first ceremonies, and beginning to speak of tilling new soils and casting new seed. Call a new circle together or sit within a trusted and established one and count the coups, publish the failures and shortcomings, lament the losses and own the gains of the year. This can be a time to name the names of those who were born to us and those who made the long canoe journey into the western medicine mystery—a time to stand up, step out, come out, and shine as farmers of our lives in the Divine Garden of the Natural World. Our endeavors have served us well, or not so well, but we accept, forgive, refocus, renew, raise a voice in prayer and gratitude, and keep "being breathed."

The feasting and fasting occasions and the year that made them give us the new stories to tell, new songs to sing, and the new dances to dance in the long winter nights to come. This is the time to gather close around a fire and tell the stories until the children lay in slumber on floor or lap and the fire burns low, casting long shadows on wall, forest, beach, wigwam, or teepee.

The seeds of our endeavors and harvests stand in balance and harmony, prepared to enter the coming Quiet Time and mindfully enter upon and within the personal and collective high winter ceremonies of the Quiet Time and the time of firing the seeds of *inspiration* for a new year!

This cycle and walk around the beautiful Mother Earth and Father Sky-Sun is completing. Thus concludes this sweat lodge ceremony of life. Thank you for your words, prayers, attention, your blood, sweat and tears...You are released. You are released to make new steps, balanced and harmonious steps into this new year and all coming new years.

Blessings, now and forever more...

Shewendagzewinodopi...a blessing has been visited upon us here.

The Harvest and Picking "In a Good Way"

Earth Ceremonies of the Gathered Plant, Leaf, Stem, Seed, and Root

The picking and gathering activities of all seasons are remarkable and important, but the autumn harvests of the just completed growing season are the final preparations for this winter, and are often prized and stored against drought, famine, or lack, for many years to come. Prayers, intention, labor, and growth-supporting warmth and moisture have produced the fruit, nut, and vegetable...green that feeds all beings, beings such as ourselves, the four-legged, those that swim, fly, slither, and crawl that eat more than water, minerals, air, and light, as do the seed beings. Most of these plant beings also produce valuable medicine seeds, roots, leaves, sap, milk, and stems. The abundantly produced, gathered, and stored *skebyak*, the green beings, and their seeds will feed, clothe, and house many; they will provide materials for tools and, most importantly, they will provide instructive stories, which will be told during the long winter nights and in the coming years. The genetic imprint of each seed nourishes our bodies and contributes intelligence from the natural world, the elemental directions and colors, the physical cycles of other living things—composted materials of all kinds, electric solar emanations, the life carrying vibration of the water beings, fire charges from the fire beings, manifold Spirit breaths carried by the ethers, winds, and air beings, and minerals released by the rock beings.

The abundance of the autumn harvest is a life metaphor, which speaks of and demonstrates a mutual and respectful interaction representing the basic giving-away and receiving nature of duality of Spirit as it evolves out of our minds and the mind of the Creator, assuming and manifesting in physical form, life incarnate.

And this physical form itself will change its face many times and undergo a multitude of shifts. The cycles of life suggest many possibilities of being. Spirit may once again enliven a two-legged form, or the intelligence may elect to merge with the water beings; sprout as a grass, shrub, or tree; run with the fire, air, or Wind Beings; join with the salts, crystals, or minerals; fuse with a direction, color, or animal; or dance to the heartbeat the Mother Earth. Spirit can, will, and may elect to expand concurrent knowingness with many of these beings, then as now, alive in a living world. The principle objective ceremony is that of cultivating and maintaining a mindful consciousness, endeavoring to heal that which is out of balance. Engaging in personal ritual, prayer, sacred movement, gratitude, and high intention is to honor and celebrate right relationship with ourselves and all of these beings, so that perceptions of separation with the Creator, ourselves, or anything else are narrowed, closed, and made whole...This is harvest made enduring, whole, and ongoing. Seed is what carries the harvest of wisdom, knowledge, and new life forward.

May 20, 2014, 15:00 CST

The Ceremony of Picking and Gathering "In a Good Way"

Picking and gathering have long been among humankind's primary tools for providing food. The basic nature of the sacred give-away and receive principle is the model for our approach to the plant people, the *skebyak,* and the natural world.

The plant people go a long way toward offering and providing us, the two-leggeds and others, with the physical materials we need to live life "in a good way." Plant fiber provides assorted fibers for the weaving of clothing, nets, mats, basketry, footwear, hammocks, housing, cordage, snares, and traps. The plant people share their bodies that our own might live, and their medicines by which we may maintain, heal, and restore health and balance.

The green beings hold all wisdom and knowledge. The Mother Earth and all beings that live upon and within her body have their own unique medicine ways and it is of these ways that we seek to learn the languages, uses, and songs. Our Mother is a sentient being with an evolutionary path of her own, and when sufficiently sensitized it is possible for us to feel her heartbeat through the soles of our feet and entire being.

In order for us to make orderly and honorable approaches to each living thing we must first understand ourselves, for this is what we bring forward in dialogue and intent by way of introduction. The text of *Spirit Talk* is designed to offer and provide sensitization models and histories, on identifying, arriving at, and holding appropriate thought focus, charting some designs of personal ritual and time management, suggesting structures of meaningful ceremony in the context of individual biology and life style, and observing and creatively participating in the cyclical dynamics of the seasons, to encourage song, dance, music…These are some of the ways by which we may begin to accurately and healthily track our minds, authentically and honorably present ourselves to ourselves, actually, and then to all other beings. Seriously consider these suggestions and the practices set forward in the earlier seasonal writings. Experiment with them for personal veracity, test them out, through your own Spirit Talk. Make requests and prayers for inspired and illuminated pathways.

The Direction of the West, the Physical, Medicine, and Introspection

Color: Black or dark blue

The animals often associated with this direction are the bear and the deer, however, many people find that personal affinities with each of the directions may reveal themselves differently in time. The Medicine Wheel designs offered on these pages are of a universal nature. Personal colors and animals may be added alongside the universal motifs, as contact, experience, familiarity, and intuition accrues with the seasons. This is a direction of deep return and recognition. The west receives us in our mysterious entirety.

THE HARD ROAD OF LIFE

West, the final direction in this cycle, links the physical plane—west, with the mental plane—east. This is called the hard road of life, and where it crosses the Good Red Road is where the Sacred Flowering Tree lives. That's *us*,…especially when we have walked all of the roads for we must not deny walking any of the paths. Here and now is where we can aspire to make our return to the home center and merge with the World Tree of Life.

The World Tree of Life

All of the previous teachings, labors, and observances are contributing to a profound return connection with the Spirit Dream
origins of the year, winter. With the arrival of autumn we reach a
culmination of medicines and seasons. Our harvests, the time of
gathering and picking is among the most mysterious, gathering
these secretive and familial beings, the beings of seed. We can
join our essences with theirs—our dualities, singularities, multi-
plicities, and universalities, unique and connected upon all directions of the Medicine Wheel, but especially the direction of the
west in the autumn, twilight of the year. Everything is coming
together. We begin to make ourselves ready to meet the demands
and rewards of the hard road of life walk, so that another cycle
can draw to an orderly close, be complete, rest, prepare, and fire
the new seeds with inspiration, jointly.

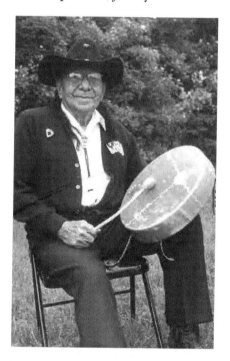

Making New Relations

Marcellus "Bear Heart" Williams, Muscogee-Creek, principle among the many gifted and loving teachers with which I have lived, generously "helped me out, Indian way." with many spoken teachings, his written word *The Wind is My Mother*, life examples, medicine experiences, energetic transmissions through osmosis and telepathy, and an unstinted sharing of his resources, connections, and his vast "Bear Heart" that saw all people without the lens of separation.

I grew up knowing of "Uncle" as a distant relation through my mother Lillian Hogue Crumbo, Muscogee-Creek. Uncle only found me when I needed him and my training began then. He was a Peyote Road man. My father, Woody Crumbo, was also a peyote man and through him I had also gone "that way." So, one day when Uncle and family drove up in Taos, New Mexico, for a peyote meeting, my house was where they came. Indian way, when there is someone from your tribe in the area, that's where you head, so sometime in the mid-1970s my close association and training with Uncle began. Friends and I poured coffee for him and his cronies, who by that time knew where he was staying. We fried his eggs and prepared the symbolic food and foods for the morning feast, which would follow the meeting that was coming up that weekend.

Picking "in a Good Way"

Picking "in a good way" was to become a teaching that would permeate my life. This teaching would influence and guide just about anything and everything that came afterward in my life. Because my trust in Uncle's medicine and confidence in his integrity and love was absolute, I was able to take on this teaching for a lifetime. I followed his direction on this, and all things, completely for I knew if any error were to be made, it would be mine for failing to follow direction, forgetting, or a lapse of willingness to be true to the teachings. I shall pass to you now, these teachings, along with a few personal relevant findings, which may help you understand. There is a lot to these teachings.

Uncle said, "First of all, don't pick when you're 'on your moon.' If it's the last day, that's okay." At that time he didn't instruct me on what to pick, why, or when—didn't need to, the lesson was on picking.

"Second, you want to fast before going out—coffee's okay.." Get some tobacco for an offering.

Take a cloth out to that spot you want to go to and lay it down. Sit down yourself for fifteen or twenty minutes, so the plants can get to know you. Think about and tell the plants who you are and what you want. Ask if some of them would be willing to "help you out" by giving their life and coming home with you. After a while, when it feels right or you just find yourself getting up, standing, and walking around, make the tobacco offering. We say, "put down some tobacco." Don't pick the first ones that you see and don't clean out a tribe or family by taking too much or everything. Do not take the Grandmother or Grandfather plants.

Use no metal, only the hands, a rock or bone knife. No exceptions.

Gather only what you can hold and make frequent trips to the cloth. If something drops leave it on the ground. It gives a mixed message to the plant, which thought it was returning to the earth. Pay more attention to how much you are carrying and how carefully. Has greed, haste or inattention taken over?

Pay close attention to when it seems like you have "enough." It's a subtle message and easy to override, especially if you have come a long way or have identified a great need for this medicine.

When the "enough" message is overridden, the pick will get tougher. You will develop a feel for this message. Picking one to three more plants is okay, if you just can't help yourself, but really try to stop there. Abuse of the plant beings can result in unknown and probably unacknowledged difficulties. You don't want to do this. The foremost and most benign of results could possibly be that you would forget, and picking would not be for you.

When you have "enough" stop, sit down, and enjoy the day. Be grateful and say thanks for the giveaways. Wrap up and tie the bundle securely. Once home, spread and dry the plants in an airy but not windy, closed, or too hot environment. A table is good. It is not in my tradition to tie and hang plants upside down for drying. Turn them several times in the next few days and when they are completely dry, store in paper or cloth sacks so they can breathe.

These are living treasures that can assist you and others in the restoration of balance and harmony. You are continuing upon your great life journey and taking on the possibility of strong and helpful medicine friends. Your approach has been good. Remain open, loving, and mindful of care and need wherever it may be found, or if it finds its way to your door, through a friend, letter, or phone. You will probably be the first beneficiary of this action. Your own personal need will most likely need to be treated and this is good. Treat yourself first. The relationship and benefit between yourself and the plant beings will grow in knowledge and trust with healing results.

SPIRIT TALK

The test: I once identified a chronic but minor condition I had previously been successful in treating. I was out of the medicine and planned a trip to the hills to pick. Everything was in place, I fasted, and was not on my moon. I set out early and drove quite a distance to a place where I had seen the plants growing, had tobacco, the cloth, everything. Everything was going well. It was a beautiful, dry, and clear day in the foothills and the air was pungent with sagebrush. Everything was in readiness and I sat down to rest, enjoy, and do my Spirit Talk. And then, when I got up to pick I only saw one or two plants where I was sure there had been more a few days earlier. I wasn't sure what to do, after all, the drive, the preparation, and the need had been considerable. I thought "maybe, since my need is great and everything has been prepared, it would be okay to take these." The great lie. Oh, my. I was so ashamed that I was even considering going against what I had been taught. But, fortunately my trust in Uncle's direction was strong enough medicine to bring me to my senses and cut off the willful thoughts, allowing me to resettle in the loving teachings. I knew if something was going to go wrong in this story it would not be due to Uncle's teaching but me, and I did not want that to happen.

"This is the bite we survive only if we are strong enough to endure the pain of allowing ourselves to be taught something we've long not known or refused to know."—Eric Francis (planetwaves.net).

I said, "Okay," packed up my gear, and laid down for a rest. Upon arising I was surrounded by a field of the plants and flowers where previously there had been few, and I was so happy I had done the right thing. Then I picked and have been picking ever since with many more "miraculous" stories. That's the way it is with me.

SPIRIT TALK

May I suggest how you might decide where to begin thinking? Books contain a vast repository of knowledge that each of us can and must turn to in the absence of a physical teacher. Start by reading an herb book (or books) that lists complaints and plant remedies and find one that matches up with a minor condition of your own. There will be many listings but read through them all. Establish a mindful and intuitive-recognizable mind, heart, body, and spirit screen in advance of the read. Make notes of which plants, if any, piqué your interest, especially if the plants grow in your area. Go over the material again. Give it some time. Engage in Spirit Talks with the material in the book. See how you feel.

Go out, sit, and look at the plants. Put down some tobacco and don't even think about picking anything.

When it comes time to go out and see what happens: make your Spirit Talk.

Prayerfully speak to each plant, greet them, and ask that they overlook any pain or discomfort you may cause, explain again why you have come and respectfully request that they might accompany you home, and help you in your life.

Speak from your heart, your innermost being, for there is no other way. Assemble your full integrity and speak of your heart-felt need. The needs you speak of at this time may surprise you by being different from what you had planned to speak. Your spirit now comes forward. This is your integrity. Speak it; listen to what it has to say.

At some point, a small breeze may waft through your picking area. Allow it to caress your cheek. Again, you are noticing every little thing…will you remember that the Wind Beings carry spirits to the Spirit World? This wind is coming to the assistance of those plants, who are now in active transition. It should be a gentle breeze but if it is not, immediately review yours and any companion picker's tools. Ideally you know and are in agreement about not using metal tools and the presence of any active moon-time activities. Stop and visit every person present in an effort to determine why a strong or erratic wind has come up. Should an error be present, immediately curb all picking by everyone. These breezes, even the winds, will make your heart feel good for they are demonstrating the interconnectedness of all living things.

Later, when the medicine is asked to be useful or the to be food eaten, the basket woven, the wild teas brewed and served, the home smudged with sage or sweet grass,…all picked "in a good way," this beautiful day will be recalled to live in our memory once more. Take the time to remember how the sun looked, how the air smelled, and the season. Upon completing these medicine journeys, mindfully return all stems, flowers, roots, or seeds to the Mother with gratitude and a pinch of corn meal or tobacco. This is but one of the myriad ways by which we recognize, create, maintain, restore, and celebrate harmony, balance, and unity with ourselves, the Creator, and all of our relations. By such simple and homely earth ceremonies does our world keep going "in a good way."

Thank you, Creator for all of the gifts, the gift of my life, and the lives of all. *Aho!*

HARVEST RECIPES

For Feasting and Circle Gatherings

Lillian Faye's Pecan Pralines

2 cups sugar
1 tsp. soda
1 cup buttermilk
Pinch of salt

Use a large kettle, the mixture foams up in cooking. Cook all above ingredients briskly, stirring frequently for 5 minutes, or until candy thermometer registers 210° degrees F.

2 tbsp. butter
2 1/2 cups whole pecans

Stir a little more and add the above ingredients. Stir continuously for 5 minutes or until candy thermometer registers 230° degrees F., or until syrup dropped into water forms a very soft ball.

Remove from heat. Stand by until mixture cools slightly. Beat until thick and creamy and drop by spoonful on waxed paper.

Lillian's Lemon Pie

Make and bake a pie shell in advance, and cool. (Just use more Crisco than any recipe calls for and you're good!)

Pie Filling

1 cup sugar
1/3 cup sugar
1/4 tsp. salt
2 cups boiling water
2 egg yolks, beaten
1tbsp. butter
1 large lemon, juice and grated rind

Mix dry ingredients and add boiling water. Boil one minute, stirring constantly.

Place over hot water or double boiler, and add egg yolks and butter; cook until thick.

Add lemon juice and rind and pour into cooked pie shell; cover with meringue and brown in preheated oven at 350° degrees F.

Meringue

2 egg whites
2 tbsp. sugar
1/8 tsp. salt
1/4 tsp. vanilla

Beat egg whites and salt until stiff but not dry; add all other ingredients; spread on top of pie filling, being sure it touches crust all around.

Gram's Fried Chicken

Now, Gram went out in the yard with her wire chicken-foot catcher, chased, and caught a chicken near every day of her life. After a fire was built in the stove and before breakfast was started, she had milked the cow, killed, scalded, plucked, cleaned, and cut up a chicken and set it to fry. The stove was hot from the fire she had started earlier, so she set the chicken to fry in bacon grease and made breakfast.

Now, the girls, one of which was my mother Lillian Faye, had food to carry for school lunch.

Grandmother Hogue's Wild Grape Dumplings

(Good Fall Medicine to Feed the Sweetness of Life)

Wild grape dumplings are one of the staple sweets of the Muscogee Creek Indians of Oklahoma. These dumplings were enjoyed by most of the tribes who were originally from the Southeast United States. Fox grapes, as they are also called, are actually a rare fall treat for the rains can be scarce throughout the early fall, drying up the grapes, leaving only the climbing vine stems for boys to cut and pretend smoke. But when the grapes do "make" they can result in a delicious broth when sweetened with honey or sugar and thickened by the flour dumplings. As a young girl, I thought Gram's dumplings floating on top of the sweet soup were the best dessert I ever had.

Since many years can go by without a grape harvest, resourceful cooks now use purple grape juice and add in a handful of concord or red grapes for color, texture, and flavor. Cherry juice and fruit also make a good dish. Substitute any fruit of choice for a delicious sweet treat.

Gram was an old-school cook whose measures were by the hand-full, the teacup, scoop, pinch, and smidgen. Her butter was measured in walnut-size pieces. Her ham and bacon came out of the smokehouse, vegetables from the garden, and household water was drawn from the spring and carried by bucket to the house. The Hogue's were a farm family who never had running water, electricity, gas, or a car.

Gram and Poppa showed me how to live with grace, hard work, gratitude, and fun in the Black Jack hills of Oklahoma.

Gram's Dumpling Recipe

2 cups flour
1 tsp. baking powder
3 tbsp. shortening
1 egg
Salt to taste

Water to mix, roll very thin on a floured board, and cut in triangles. Lower the dumplings gently, one by one, into the simmering fruit juice broth, cover and cook until done, about 10 minutes.

Gram's Wild Grape Broth

Pick and clean the grapes of leaves, stems, and tendrils, wash and cover with water.
Simmer for 15–20 minutes, covered, sweeten to taste depending on the amount of water used, usually about 1/2 cup of sugar.

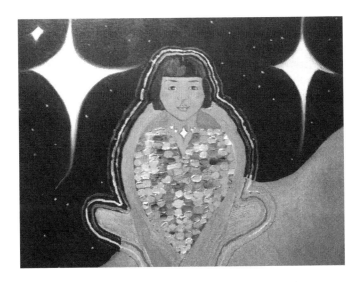

The Circle Gathering, Part 1

The circle gathering is recognized as first ceremony. There is a long tradition of persons gathering to parlay, celebrate, mark, and honor with dance; accuse, adjudicate, and mediate; provide direction and information; inform and publish; raise energy; be born, heal, and die, and to initiate and negotiate important, witnessed thresholds, while walking the axial passages and pastures of the seasons.

The circle gathering may be any of these things but it will also be its own "thing," unpredictable despite agenda, uncontrollable by nature, and unbelievably valuable as an arena within which summoned, interested, involved, or committed members may take up the wooden staff of integrity and speak their truths as they know them to be, occasionally surprising even themselves when the truths begin to break the surface of the waters and emotions reveal the rocks and rifts upon which their frail crafts sail.

The circle gathering's potent aura, gathered from personal vibrational frequencies, consciously or unconsciously connects and infuses the sitter, dancer, or speaker with core earthly and solar resonances. This core column of energy seats and channels all intention that comes near, within, or even hears about it with the ear, extra senses, or talk, and amplifies and broadcasts, to a certain degree, all that happens within. However, highly confidential, familial, tribal, or governmental council talks will take energetic steps to secure the ordinarily permeable outer membrane or outer circle, warranting a greater degree of confidentiality. Teachings such as these bring privacy, in a privacy challenged world, back into our hands, honorably garnering and gathering our most self-respecting instincts to survive and then to flourish. So it is with first ceremony, which we will now call council or talking circle. The stick is in *our* hands.

There is no wrong way to sit in council but certain local protocols, ground rules, and precedents will exist...Inform yourself of them. Courteous and respectful behavior is always desirable. Certain mores of behavior will draw on cultural precedent and others will be simple and flexible. Two universal precepts ruling all important circle gatherings are the absolute sobriety of each attendant and the attendants' confidence that they will be given ample time to speak once they have been awarded the staff of integrity, or talking stick—to rise, to hold the floor, and begin to speak their truth. The talking circle will most assuredly be the finest, most trustworthy, safe, and supportive opportunity available, probably ever, by which to confidently, or unconfidently, step up and "raise a voice."

An individual, scheduled or spontaneous gathering of two is a meeting, and three or more persons begin to form a group. From this point on, pay attention to every little thing. This is always good council, but attention to detail will support your recording and recollection of the important spoken word in an invaluable way. Hone conversational skills, such as extending affirmations when asking what the other person(s) heard you say and asking permission to relay what you heard. Courteously allow corrections and additions to be spoken, without interruption. Endeavor to converse, listen, and respond in turn, not react. Speak to what was said and save the defensive response for when there is more information. Remember the old game of Gossip? Why fall prey to that old saw? Form agreements to be as forthcoming and clear as possible, striving mutually for interactive and accurately perceived comprehension.

Local precept, style, and tradition will build foundation and structure to house life's most precious commodity—our selves, community, family, friends, associates, and the larger world. Examples of how various talking circles might form and the formats they might take under consideration will follow.

The Circle Gathering, Part 2

The circle gathering or talking circle was an integral part of the traditional women's way teachings that I held energy for and taught for twenty-eight years, under the auspices of the Moon Circle Teachings Group. At the end of the twenty-eighth year, the imperative to communicate the women's ways, as delivered to me in Spirit form twenty-eight years earlier, quietly and unobtrusively melted back into the twenty-eight day cycle of the women's moon time, or period of monthly blood flow.

During that teaching time I served the public with ceremony and ritual opportunities, committed women's medicine groups, traveled, wrote, painted, and spoke of the blood mysteries and the women's way to vision quest and forge a balanced feminine empowerment through the sacred charge offered by our bodies and gender definition.

The talking circle was, and remains, the centerpiece activity for any gathering. The importance of the circle cannot be over-emphasized. It functions as the organ, blood, bone, viscera, and breath of the marriage column, and the circle itself, defines, contains, and surrounds the column as a skin, shield, or membrane. The marriage column is where the Mother Earth and the Father Sky-Sun, our elemental parents, meet and mingle with us in the sacred circle, encouraging us to speak our clear and unclouded truths, within the protective viscera of the creative birth canal, truths we knew before the separation anxieties arose and we began to forget. Here in the circle we begin to remember, and to reveal, ourselves to ourselves and to others.

The Circle Gathering, Part 3

The circle format, which works well for me, is permeated with the spirits of our elemental parents and is superimposed over the energetics of the Medicine Wheel. The selected circle area is cleaned and cleared with the assistance of the sage beings, whose smoke serves to dispel any negative energies, and the sweetgrass beings, who give their bodies and essence to bless the cleared spaces and fill them with love until we find something else to take that place. This blessing forestalls any feelings of too-rapid loss or abandonment when things leave quickly, and it fills spaces with love that might otherwise be open and vulnerable to roaming opportunistic spirit entities seeking shelter. This is done before any guest enters the area, places objects, or sits down. During this process a circle, with a doorway in the east, is naturally drawn and then *may* be emphasized with a cornmeal or tobacco line. If the circle is not physically drawn it should be thought or prayed in place by the facilitator or helper. This is a living altar. It will later be disassembled, swept away, and returned to the Mother.

For privacy's sake and to help insure clear attention, provide the attendees with another room for cell phones—silenced, and iPads.

Ask all those attending to clear the evening, enabling activities to proceed into the night undisturbed by schedules. This time is for all of us, alone.

After everyone has entered the circle and been seated on the floor or ground, they can be

"fanned-off" with sage and sweetgrass. Some people like to do this outside the circle.

After greeting the club, sodality, sisterhood, baptismal group, moon circle, drum circle, twelve-step or other group with serious intentions, the evening is opened with a prayer and the talking stick, as a symbol of integrity, will be introduced. Each person will be invited to stand, call their name, and say why they are present, and they are welcome to speak their crooked, or straight, truth in the renewal circle. Each speaker will signal their finish by saying, "That's the way it is with me," whereupon they will walk the staff to the next person to their sunwise (clockwise) left, pass it to the standing person, and return to their seat, walking all the way around the circle, sunwise. The talking stick will visit each person. If anyone elects not to speak they may stand, receive the stick, say, "That's the way it is with me," pass the stick on to the next person, and sit.

There is no telling how this will go. Some people need to visit unity to get a clear vision of their duality issues and blessings; others need to temporarily depart from unity to gain perspective from the sidelines.

A closing prayer will help restore a sense of balance and harmony to each person, no matter how jagged or smooth their talk has been. This is *very* important. People *cannot* be left in disarray or off of their center by the trusting act of daring to speak their truth. This is why the circle is earlier "mellowed" by the purifying smokes, making this a safe place.

If there are matters of interest, teaching, or schedule to discuss, it can now be done now. The assembled group will be reminded that no talk will leave the circle.

Then, an expression of gratitude is expressed and offered to the Medicine Wheel elemental parents, the directions and colors, the helper Spirits—the custodians on the land and in the hearts of each and every participant, remembering the blessings of Creation, self, and the fellowship experienced. The group then prepares to calmly stir with the womb-circle-birth column, to feel their fingers and toes, stretch, and come back into the body, for we will have moved much more deeply into Spirit than we realized. Now, we begin to rise and leave the womb, through the birth canal to emerge, renewed, refreshed, purified, and reborn to self. Look into the eyes of the others and see the beauty, calm, and joy,…and yours reflected back at you.

A visit to a well-prepared circle gathering is truly first ceremony, as when the world was new. Allow yourself to "be breathed."

A potluck feast has been organized and is now offered. If someone knows how to prepare an offering plate, that can be done now,…another prayer to the beings which are giving their lives so that life might go on "in a good way."

Eat and feel good. Do you need to prepare a plate to take to someone waiting at home?

Go home carefully. Make yourself visible from your deep journey into Spirit. Move slowly, be breathed, and don't feel like you must speak to or answer any questions, no matter how loving and well-intentioned they are, at this time. Simply smile, give a kiss or a hug, and say, "It went great! But not now honey, maybe later? Tell me about *your* evening…" Be nice. Your loved ones may just want to know, but they may be feeling a little left out. You will know what to do…

That's the way Sweet Medicine goes.

The Circle Gathering, Part 4

The Spirit Plate, Alive in a Living World

The Spirit plate makes our recognition and gratitude visible to the beings who are making a gift of their seed history, and when properly addressed they can become actively involved in an ongoing life path through other agents, namely ourselves. Their seed histories, with cultural family trees grounded in the natural world that make contributions of inestimable value and tensile strength to the DNA of any bonding entity, are at least as hugely long and venerable as ours.

Most of these connections and contributions are beyond our ken, but heartfelt gestures of gratitude and respect for these living things are ours to express through remembering our connections to the best of our ability—where and when they lived and grew, who harvested them, how they were handled and for what purpose and by whom. The questions are always, what do we have to do that these things will live?

The Spirit plate is prepared by selecting very small and representative pieces of each feast food on the table. This is done immediately prior to the feast. The seed, meat, fluid, fruit, vegetable, and grain particles are mindfully collected with the left, offering hand, taken outside, and offered with a prayer of recognition and gratitude to the Master of All Breath that their essence returns and eats first.

I like to raise the plate and turn it to the seven directions, lastly approaching the Mother four times before lowering the plate to the earth. I reenter, a feasting prayer for all of the gifts is offered, and the eldest persons come forward to eat first.

Shewen dagzewin! A blessing is visited upon us this day!

July 6, 2014

Bringing It All Together

The harvest. The harvest can be many things. It is all things, collected and organized along particular lines of choice, interest, necessity, whim…lines of interest, twisted with plant particle, animal hair, possibly threads of metal, saturated with dyes of mineral and plant origin...lines of intellectual, spiritual, political, and emotional thought forms brought together upon the looms and interlocking webs of flow charts, projection and production models, reflecting abundance and lack upon scales suited to the relative interpretation of survival, strong survival, building, and flourishing potentials.

The harvest represents hidden and visible influences. The harvest represents the gathering together of chaotic and random natural forces linked with intelligence, specific intent, happenstance, vigilance, and applied skill. The harvest represents what has come forward, what is present in the granaries of measured resource for today and tomorrow. The harvest is the belly that the arms and spine of effort have fed. The harvest has brought forward the new seeds.

At this time it is good to study deeply upon the methodologies that brought us to this place, how well they worked or did not work. The well-evaluated harvest suggests viewing new and outmoded partnerships, relative nutritional values, and variable strength levels of the incoming material. Many strengths and vigors are in strong flow, surging even. Some strengths are diminished or exhausted, and some strengths will reveal themselves as having maintained structure and timbre throughout the past year. All are charted, cooked, shaped, or woven to reveal larger pictures, garments, tools, dishes, or understandings.

Harvest feasts, celebrations, and ceremonies are essentially designed to commemorate effort, to affirm, partner with, and initiate the formation of new brain matrices, which will carry us successfully forward through the winter firing ceremonies and another cycle.

The strategies of each season are specific and interrelated, making it possible to plan and diagram the passage of any given season in the larger context of a year, to the best of *our* ability. But perhaps the most viable plan would include an update of our original tools, the brain, heart, body, and integrated spirit. It would include forming a renewed and updated brain matrix, a healthy body, and a broadened feeling capacity out of this season's unification gains.

Formulating an Updated Brain Matrix

As the wisdom and purity qualities of winter were opposite and intimately connected to the love and innocence qualities of the south by polarity, the introspective west is opposite and yet similarly intimately connected to the mental qualities of the east. These polarities exert great balancing and harmonizing influences upon one another. Spring and fall are twilights of the seasons. The spring twilight is Earth emergent and the fall twilight is Earth returning. They share the fires and have equivalent and inseparable values. The east and the west "arms" of the Medicine Wheel "embody" the quality of balance between the mind and body, while the north and south axis can be viewed as the energetic spine, or chakra system, which embodies the quality of harmony.

The words "balance" and "harmony" are the crosshairs and sacred flowering center of the w(holy) Medicine Wheel construct. They, and therefore we, are part and parcel and inextricably incorporated into, within, and upon this encircling Sun-Moon-Earth-Star-Seasonal Wheel of Life.

The resultant potential for the seasonal, or even moment to moment, rebuilding or contribution to this central-flowering brain matrix is ever present and attainable through intent, selected daily activities, and interests. These interests represent yet another marriage of compatible opposites representing many of the commensurate and relatively balanced qualities and quantities of duality. Most physical activities that employ arms, the brain, and the spinal column, present opportunities to bring the left and right together in the center and create the potential for a very new creative action. Sports of all kinds, swimming, knitting, yoga, reading, thinking, looking and seeing, keyboard use, art, dance and music creations (choose your own) are some of the balanced activities, which can gradually or spontaneously bring the conscious qualities of balance and harmony together in a unified field with resultant contributions to the growth of a more vital brain matrix.

This is a true conscious interaction of positive evolutionary thrust, fused and anchored within the spinal-arm axis and seated in the central home of an increasingly unified awareness. Focused and well-intentioned movements in personal concert with the new seeds, the powers of the natural world, and the first gifts can bring every person into a finer attunement with self, all of Creation, and the Great Mystery as brought to us by the Master of All Breath.

FALL EQUINOX

September 21–22

The medicine direction of the west has arrived, bringing the moving inward time. Harvest also comes and with it some of the gifts we will carry inward for the all-important "time of introspection."

This season of the Medicine Wheel...carefully inspect, count, and look to recognize and gain as much information, inspiration, and energy as you are able from these seeds, which carry much import. Only we can decipher and correctly interpret our personal harvest.

This is the time to gift the seeds, fruits, and herbs with gratitude and unconditional love. It begins with mindfulness, and from there each of us may design our own personal harvest ceremonies, which may also include song, prayers, dance, and feasting.

Recall this past spring and tell the story to life...and the coming winter, who will accept and carry these seeds in her belly to give birth to the next planting season. These seeds will encode your stories within their histories and say how it was/is with us. A part of their healthy lives is contingent upon the quality of our participation as co-Creators.

As we face the west, let us remember and accept that the east-spring-planting season is at our back. When we are not sure how to proceed, or what to say, we have but to ask and to be willing for the power of the direction to provide inspiration for fertile and gracious thoughts and words.

Sometimes we wonder who all of the other "theys" are. The directions can be asked for information also. At your daily sunrise ceremony you may ask, "Grandfather, what would you have me know this day?" Accept the first thought that comes to you. In this way, we take the mindful steps of building spiritual muscle and capital. Reflect on that first thought throughout the day... test it out. It's up to us to build these roads and pathways, asking, is it true or not? What more is there to know or carry forward in my life? Not knowing is an outcome of our perceived separation from the Creator and is so much more painful than knowing. For in knowing, things can begin to move into dynamic change, and in not knowing...too many things are managed in a way that they remain hidden, or aggressively in mind and difficult to dislodge, evolve, or release.

The directions, Sun, Moon, plants, waters, winds, fires, stones... all knowledge is held in the Natural World—the free university of natural wisdom and intelligence.

Make application and attend daily. Do your homework. Ask questions, pay the dues and tuitions of awareness and gratitude. Tell everyone who your teachers are and what your alma mater is. Why love her, him, and them less? Why forget and place all others first?

Go *team Creation!*

Dawn Woman

Dawn @ the Ranch

SPIRIT TALK

The only and best path we have to the restoration, maintenance, and growth of our fullest potential sensitization lies in rediscovering and grounding our highest intentions, and thereby beginning to close the perceptions of separation with the Creator and beginning to recognize and experience ourselves as seed co-Creator's, though our willingness to engage in Spirit Talks with our essential selves, our elemental parents, the Natural World, and the seasons.

Many helpers, systems, guides, messages, practices, religions, and traditions will be found to be of core essential assistance, inspiration, illumination, and support on an individual's journeys toward and within the restoration and the continual renewal of balance and harmony. The culmination of these paths then finds its natural destination within the unity path—the spiritual evolutionary path of humanity, drawn out of and for the fullest honoring and manifestation of the Creative duality principal, now in place upon the Mother Earth.

The unity path brings forward the most evolved and individuated gifts of mind, heart, body, and spirit of the individual soul, in preparation for our successful launch as universal citizens, in the highest and best possible Ways.

Many are the paths but the first, most beautiful, enduring, and visibly tangible of the Creative gifts lie within and upon the wisdom libraries of the natural world, the ethers, our Grandmother the Moon, the Star Beings, our Mother the Earth and our Father the Sky-Sun, and all who live upon and within this miraculous world.

Be breathed and know life.

Aho!

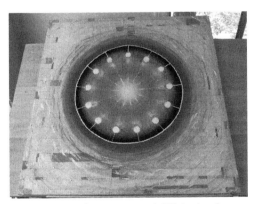

The thirteen moons have been traversed. We begin the new seed cycle.

GLOSSARY

Aho!	It is good! (strong affirmative)
Ahora	(Spanish)Now
Bama mine	See you later
Bodewadmin	Potawatomi
Bomgék	Winter
Bozho nikan	Hello, my bone (a traditional greeting)
Demén	Strawberry
Dgwagék	Autumn
Ehe	Yes
Gishget	Autumn leaves turning yellow
Gon	Snow
Guna gish pi	The Place of the Morning Star
Migwech, wewene, kiche migwech	
	Thank you, thank you very much
Minén	Blueberry
Mitakweasin	All my relations
Mkedémen	Blackberry
Mnokmek	Spring
Mskomén	Raspberry
Ni je na	How are all of you

Nibnék	Summer
Noden	Wind
Sé ma	Tobacco man
Shewendagzewinodopi	A blessing is visited on us here
Skebyak	The Green Beings
Wabaksekwe	Dawn Woman

SUGGESTED READINGS

Estes, Clarissa Pinkola. *Women Who Run with the Wolves: Myths and Stories of the Wild Woman Archetype.* New York: Ballentine Books, 1992

Hill, Ruth Beebe. *Hanto Yo: An American Saga.* New York: Doubleday, 1979

Neihardt, John G. *Black Elk Speaks: Being a Life Story of a Holy Man of the Oglala Sioux.* New York: William Morrow and Company, 1932

Prechtel, Martin. *Long Life, Honey in the Heart: A Story of Initiation and Eloquence from the Shores of a Mayan Lake.* New York: Jeremy P. Tarcher/Putnam, 1999.

Storm, Hyemeyohsts. *Seven Arrows.* New York: Harper and Row, 1972.

Williams, Marcellus "Bear Heart," with Molly Larkin. *The Wind is My Mother: The Life and Teachings of a Native American Shaman.* New York: Random House, 1996.

Ywahoo, Dhyani. *Voices of Our Ancestors: Cherokee Teachings from the Wisdom Fires.* Boston: Shambala Publications, 1987.